Jennifer Meek is a qualified nutritionist and also has a degree in microbiology. In addition to writing, she teaches science.

IMMUNE POWER

HEALTH AND THE IMMUNE SYSTEM

JENNIFER MEEK

An OPTIMA Book

© Jennifer Meek, 1990

First published in 1990 by
Macdonald Optima, a division of
Macdonald & Co. (Publishers) Ltd

A member of Maxwell Macmillan Pergamon Publishing Corporation

British Library Cataloguing in Publication Data

Meek, Jennifer
    Immune power.
    1. Medicine.   Immunology
    I. Title
    616.079
    ISBN 0-356-17138-8

Macdonald & Co. (Publishers) Ltd
Orbit House
1 New Fetter Lane
London
EC4A 1AR

Typeset in Ehrhard by Leaper & Gard Ltd, Bristol

Printed and bound in Great Britain by
The Guernsey Press Co. Ltd., Guernsey, Channel Islands.

CONTENTS

PREFACE

Good health is rarely achieved by chance. To keep it, we have to maintain a good biochemical balance. All disease, after all, can be traced back to some chemical disturbance in the body, and that imbalance may be caused by any one of a combination of factors, such as infectious agents, genetic faults, environmental poisons, unbalanced nutrient intake, emotional conflicts, or a whole host of other potential enemies.

Traditionally, immunology has dealt with our defences against bugs which cause disease, but with our ever-increasing knowledge of how the body works, this has been broadened to include ways in which the body defends itself against many other problems encountered during life. Life has many ingredients, some are good and others are bad, but essentially, life is for living, for learning, for loving, for achieving and for enjoying and no one wants to waste more time than they have to being sick.

We all underestimate the wisdom of our body and often ignore the body's needs, instead attending to our superficial wants, yet when the body is out of tune due to improper nutrition or unbalanced chemistry, its performance is less reliable, less capable and its appearance deteriorates.

Many years ago, as an undergraduate at Reading University, I was inspired by the immune system. It struck me as an impressive set-up: a personal survival kit, a self-repair outfit, a personal Ministry of Defence and a refuse disposal department all rolled into one. Perhaps because it couldn't be pinned to a specific organ and was spread in many forms throughout the body, it had an enigma which made its study interesting.

My interest continued whilst doing postgraduate research at Sussex University and Bristol Medical School, but it wasn't until I went to work abroad, living in what was classed as a Third World country, that the links between the condition of the immune system and dietary or environmental imbalances became obvious.

The immune system has to deal with whatever we put into our bodies. Whatever we put in will have an effect – either good or bad. It has certain requirements, necessary for the fulfilment of the tasks it needs to perform, and without them it cannot do the work properly. Many people, who have initially come to me for nutritional advice, have also become enthusiastic about experimenting with changes in food and lifestyle in order to improve mental or physical performance, mood, behaviour or resistance to disease. The scales of health are constantly shifting throughout life, so there is no single formula which will work for everyone all of the time, but it is never too early or too late to start improving your health and your life.

There are still many body processes that we do not and may never fully understand but, in the light of present knowledge, this book is an attempt to explain the immune system in very simple terms and to help readers to try to restore their own vital balance by pointing out some immune enemies and ways of avoiding or compensating for them. We cannot avoid all threats to the immune system, but we can lessen the load.

The growing interest in protecting our environment can only have beneficial effects as environmental pollution does adversely affect our health. It is important that we all care enough to feel personally involved. We are all on this earth together! To stay healthy, not only do we have to look after our external environment but we must also take care of our personal internal environments. We are all made up of cells, each with their own functions and needs. If we can maintain our cells in health and vigour, good health, vitality and longevity should follow.

I should like to thank Ruth and Ken Pike for spending a lot of their time typing up this script, Poole General Hospital for allowing me to use their postgraduate library, colleagues at work for bending timetables around 'the book', and friends and family for their support and encouragement. We are all indebted to the many people who spend years of their lives researching specific areas of immunology and medicine in their search for tomorrow's miracles and their attempts to prevent, alleviate or cure human sickness. Thanks to their work we can accumulate knowledge and so learn how to increase our immune power, our resistance to disease, our ability to heal and our enthusiam for living and being well.

I
HOW ARE YOU?

This is a very common question that we have probably all been asked more times than we can remember. Usually, we do not even bother to think about what the question means; the answer is automatic and something like 'Fine thank you. How are you?', regardless of how we really feel. The other relatively common reply lists a whole series of problems and ailments, so that the questioner wishes he had not asked in the first place.

HOW DO YOU REALLY FEEL?

- Do you lack energy, always feeling more tired than you think you should?
- Do you find it difficult to concentrate and to be interested and enthusiastic about life?
- Are you overweight?
- Are you overweight, and stay that way no matter how much you seem to count calories?
- Are you underweight although you eat a lot? Does it seem that you can eat what you like and not get fat?
- Do you get a lot of vague aches and pains?
- Do you often get common infections like colds, sore throats or thrush?
- Are you unhappy?
- Do you sleep badly?
- Are you often tense, irritable and cannot let go and relax?
- Do you already have a medical condition that is pulling you down?
- Do you feel great and want to stay that way for all your life if possible?

If you have answered 'Yes' to any of these questions and are willing to do something positive about it, you will probably find this book interesting and informative.

The public answer needs to be brief, but, in private, ask yourself this question frequently, and be honest with yourself, for your answers will provide clues to the effectiveness of your immune system. The immune system is an essential key with which we can unlock many secrets of health, vitality and longevity. It is a key which for thousands of years we did not even realise we had.

LONGEVITY AND THE IMMUNE SYSTEM

Your fighting force

The immune system is what fights off all the bugs – bacteria, viruses, fungi and protozoa – that we come across daily and those that we come across more rarely. Bugs are part of natural living; some do us harm, others help us, but the important factor is that we, not the bugs, are in control.

If we can maintain a strong, active, efficient immune system we are less likely to die from a disease caused by any of these bugs. We are also less likely to suffer from autoimmune diseases – diseases in which the immune system mistakenly reacts against some part of the body. We can be ill less often for less days of our lives. In short, a healthy immune system will keep us looking and feeling younger and living longer.

Your internal housekeeper

The immune system does all the housework around the body. It gets rid of the rubbish that accumulates during the process of living. It disposes of all the dead cells and bugs and, in true Womble fashion, its members patrol the body picking up all the rubbish.

If you think of the body rather like a house or a car, it is easy to visualise that if it is kept clean, tidy and well maintained, both inside and out, it will look better and last longer than if it is neglected. A rotten, rusty, old car is a sad sight in comparison to its well main-tained, vintage counterpart.

Pamper your immune system and aim to keep it in mint condition.

Your time keeper

The immune system has a regulatory role to play in brain function and hormone secretion. Both these play a very obvious part in the rate at which we age. Some 50 year olds look, act and have the thinking capacity of 40 year olds. Others of the same age look, act and think as if they were 65 or older. Your state of health at 50 largely determines which group you will be in.

Lifespan

A life expectancy of 70 years for man is not consistent with scientific expectation; a life span of 120 years is a more realistic figure. Although man likes to think of himself as super-intelligent and superior to the animals, he is one of the few animals studied that does not manage to live to six times the age of maturity. It has been shown many times that it is perfectly possible for animals to live for this period of time; hence an animal that matures in a matter of days can live for six times that period, assuming, of course, that it is not killed by accidents, predators, etc.

Psalm 90, verse 10 says that 'The days of our years are three score years and ten', but the verse is invariably taken out of context, and possibly the 'secret sins' mentioned in verse 8 refer to the many ways in which we have departed from a natural healthy lifestyle. We do not know. What we do know, however, is that this Psalm is known as 'A Prayer of Moses, the man of God'. In Deuteronomy 34, verse 7 we are told that Moses himself 'was an hundred and twenty years old when he died: his eye was not dim, nor his natural force abated'. It should be possible for man to live and be healthy for as long as Moses.

Mind over immunity

It is important to dispel this belief in the probability of senility or death around 70 years; as we shall see later, the mind has an amazing power over the body and the immune system. It is far easier to think yourself sick than it is to think yourself better; it is far easier to believe in the inevitability of being sick during your life than it is to believe in a miracle cure for a dreaded disease. The mind can be used as a powerful tool or a lethal weapon. Do not allow yourself to think that you will be past it at the age of 70. We do have some control over the rate at which we age and the age at which we die.

HEALTH AND THE IMMUNE SYSTEM

Our life on this planet is programmed to develop in stages. Our past enables us to grow in knowledge and to learn from our mistakes. We are able to prepare and plan for the future, but in preparing for that future we must realise that it is what we eat, think and do between, for example, 40 and 60 that determines how we feel, look and think at 70 or 80.

Probably the greatest single factor in shaping our lives is our state of health. How we cope with new experiences, challenges and problems has to be governed by the way we feel and the way we cope with how we feel. Whilst we have good health, we take it for granted. Once we have bad health, we label it as inevitable. But why leave something as important as health to chance? Life is for living, for learning, enjoying and achieving. Who wants to waste time being sick?

When you are young, or even in middle age, it is easy not to think about all those degenerative and life-threatening diseases that only happen to other people, never to you. As middle age progresses, however, all your friends seem to have one thing or another. Conversations start to have their share of age comments, like 'It's my age', 'It's getting old', 'I can't do it as well as I used to', 'I'm over the hill now', said in fun, but with a hint of truth. Even the positive 'Life begins at 40' is usually said with the tone of 'I'm saying it, but I don't believe it and neither do you.'

It is true that in some cases, where there is an inherited condition or where there has been an accident, ill health is inevitable, but in most cases we bring ill health upon ourselves by the way we eat, drink, move, think and live. We should pay as much attention to our immune systems as we do to our bank balance.

We all know that if you contribute regularly to your bank account and limit what you spend to a sensible level, depending on what you earn, you can reap the benefits of your forward planning in old age. If you neglect your bank account for 30 or 40 years, you will have only your initial assets in later life. If you make frequent withdrawals and do not bother to save, you are soon in the red and your debts could get out of control. The currency you use for your immune bank is your daily habits; the habits you accumulate over a lifetime will determine whether you are in the black or in the red when you retire.

Illness is not inevitable. If you look after your immune system, it is capable of giving good service. If you treat it with consideration, make regular contributions of healthy habits during your lifetime and restrict the unhealthy habits, so that your overall balance is always in the black, illness could be rare and relatively mild.

The history of healthy habits
Unhealthy habits have been man's greatest temptations since the Garden of Eden. Over two-and-a-half thousand years ago, in the days of the great Greek philosopher Pythagoras and the Jewish prophet Daniel, habits were linked to disease and destruction. Pythagoras is reputed to have said 'Man, by his habits, sets into motion those agencies which eventually destroy him.' This statement is timeless and can be applied today in so many ways.

SOME HEALTHY AND UNHEALTHY HABITS

Which ones do you have?

- Do you get angry easily?
- Do you avoid processed food as much as possible?
- Do you drink water from the hot tap?
- Do you get natural light (not from behind glass) on you, especially your eyes, every day?
- Do you eat a lot of fried foods (including crisps)?
- Do you avoid artificial colours and flavours in food and drink?
- Do you eat a lot of spicy, highly flavoured food?
- Do you feel competent and confident?
- Do you use the car even for short trips?
- Do you eat some fruit and vegetables every day?
- Do you get irritated easily?
- Do you enjoy life?
- Do you eat cakes and biscuits every day?
- Do you know which food supplements you need?
- Do you add sugar to your food?
- Are you satisfied with what you are doing with your life?
- Do you eat a lot of convenience food?
- Do you have a firm religious belief?
- Do you get depressed easily?
- Do you eat about 20 per cent of your food raw?
- Do you eat out in restaurants a lot?
- Do you smile and laugh often?
- Are you addicted to any food (especially tea, coffee, alcohol, sugar, wheat or chocolate)?
- Do you make friends easily?
- Do you cry or feel like crying often?
- Do you have a satisfying sex life with only one partner?
- Do you never have time to eat properly?
- Do you include a quiet period in your daily life (relaxing or meditating in silence)?
- Do you find it difficult to make or keep friends?
- Do you include oats two or three times in the weekly diet?
- Do you find it difficult to express your feelings?
- Do you sleep well?
- Do you avoid fibre-containing foods?
- Do you feel in love and loved?

- Do you suffer with sunburn often (weather permitting)?
- ○ Do you take food supplements?
- Do you feel lonely, trapped and unloved?
- ○ Do you pray or meditate?
- Are you overweight?
- ○ Do you swim once a week or more?
- Do you add salt to your food daily?
- ○ Do you eat fish once or twice a week?
- Do you use a lot of household, cosmetic or garden chemicals?
- ○ Do you include exercise (other than swimming) in your daily routine?
- Do you have a frustrating sex life?
- ○ Do you eat wholegrains other than wheat regularly?
- Do you smoke?
- ○ Do you wash frequently, but without soap?
- Do you use drugs?
- ○ Do you restrict meat to less than 2 lb per person per week?
- Do you have sex with more than one partner?
- ○ Are you happy with the shape of your body?
- Do you drink more than one measure of alcohol a day?
- ○ Do you clean your teeth after every meal?
- Do you use the pill or antidepressants?
- ○ Do you drink more than two pints of fluid a day (excluding alcoholic drinks)?
- Do you use laxatives or antacids regularly?
- ○ Do you take some mono or polyunsaturated fat every day?
- Do you use appetite suppressants, sleeping pills or pep pills?
- ○ Do you eat nuts and seeds weekly?
- Do you dwell on the day's problems in bed at night?
- ○ Do you enjoy being with your family?
- Do you live or work near electricity pylons, overhead power lines, or radio transmitters?
- ○ Do you keep animal fat to less than 15 per cent of your total diet?
- Is your daily life conducted in a noisy atmosphere?
- ○ Do you enjoy your work?
- Do you live or work in a smoky atmosphere?

Positive answers to the questions with ○ against them indicate healthy habits. Positive answers to questions with ● against them indicates a need for good habits to replace the bad ones.

Think about your habits. Are there any healthy ones which you could add to the list, or any unhealthy ones that you could perhaps modify? Habits can be boring. They are things that you do regularly, often without thinking about what you are doing. It can be interesting and fun to change them and you have a positive motive. You can avoid some unhealthy habits, boost your immune system and improve your health by switching to healthy habits.

However not all of our habits are under our direct control. For example, although we can give up smoking, it is not possible to give up passive smoking if someone in the family, a friend or a colleague smokes. Besides, we cannot avoid every attack on our immune systems. Living is a risky business and always fatal, but we can organise our lives to minimise the risks and increase the advantages.

Illness and the immune system

With an out-of-condition immune system you can expect to be ill more often and more seriously for more days of your life. There are always plenty of disease-causing bacteria, viruses, fungi and other organisms hanging around, either in the body or the environment, just waiting for their chance to attack a nice juicy human. They are part of life in this world; we cannot avoid them, but we have a system for coping with them. The details of how will follow in a later chapter, but we have several armies of immune cells which recognise these invaders, attack them and hopefully destroy them before they destroy us. If our personal immune system is overworked, inefficient or undernourished it will not be able to equip an army able to recognise the enemy and destroy it; that is when we catch a disease. How badly the illness affects us depends on how long it takes the immune system to become effective and fight back.

By maintaining our immune system in peak condition, it is, at best, possible to avoid symptoms of illness completely and, at worst, it is possible to put together an effective fighting force quickly so that the illness is less severe and does not last long.

The immune system can destroy cancer cells. We all make these cells, but keep them under control. It is when the cancer cells are formed at a rate at which the immune system cannot cope that cancer becomes a problem.

Similarly, as long as the immune system is working correctly, there is no problem with autoimmune diseases. It is only when the immune system goes wrong and does not recognise self as self any more that autoimmune diseases occur – the army starts attacking the body's own cells as well as its enemies.

Radiation and chemicals

Your immune system offers protection from radiation and from chemicals. And these days our bodies certainly have a lot of new chemicals to contend with. In fact, I would almost go so far as to say that our lifetime is the age of the chemical revolution. We use chemicals as medicines, as sprays for plants, to destroy pests, to prevent natural chemical changes like ripening or shooting. We use cosmetic chemicals, household chemicals and industrial chemicals. We even put chemicals into our food. Unfortunately our bodies have not had time to develop ways of dealing with so many new chemicals, and this is putting a strain on our immune systems.

Our exposure to radiation is also greater than it has ever been before, both from natural radiation (increased levels from sunlight and in some places from the rocks) as well as from artificial sources (medicine, industry and energy production).

WEIGHT CONTROL AND THE IMMUNE SYSTEM

The immune system even affects our weight, because it is called into action by many foods that we eat.

Anyone who has a weight problem which is not directly linked to too much or too little food consumed may well have a food sensitivity problem. When we have become sensitive to a particular food, every time it is eaten it causes the immune system to go into unnecessary battle. This sort of reaction may well start after pregnancy or after an illness, when the immune system has been modified or has had to work harder and is more liable to make mistakes.

The immune system is alerted whenever we eat cooked and processed food, but there is not the same reaction when we eat raw natural food. Eating raw food before eating cooked food lessens the load on the immune system.

If your weight is out of control because your immune army is in chaos, helping your immune system may be the key to a more shapely you.

VITALITY AND THE IMMUNE SYSTEM

To have vitality is to have enough of the right kinds of energy to perform all the necessary functions of life.

When it is overworked for any reason, the immune system snatches up all the B vitamins because it is stressed, leaving little if any to take part in the energy cycle. A vicious circle is created, leaving you with progressively less and less vitality – a sort of downward energy spiral.

With a well-tuned well-organised immune system you can benefit from greater physical energy. Not only that but, because mental energy is also sapped by a flagging immune system, getting that in tune could well improve powers of concentration and memory. Rebuilding immune power could mean getting off that downward energy spiral and climbing up the energy ladder.

WHAT AN EFFICIENT IMMUNE SYSTEM CAN DO FOR YOUR HEALTH

What are the advantages of dumping all those unhealthy habits and changing to healthy ones? How would an improved immune system affect your health?

- Symptoms of infection become less severe.
- As the immune system improves, there is less likelihood of catching colds, flu and other infections.
- Natural control over destruction of cancer cells is maximised.
- Symptoms of autoimmune diseases may be reduced.
- Natural protection from radiation is maximised.
- The aging process will be slowed down to its normal level. (We tend to accelerate it with unhealthy habits.)
- Accumulation of toxic chemicals that can cause symptoms like headaches and other vague aches and pains which sap vitality and leave you feeling tired and unenthusiastic will slowly disperse. Energy levels will then increase.
- Concentration, memory, ability to relax and sleep soundly should all improve.
- Weight problems related to the immune system should slowly even out.

In short, with a strong immune system and a positive attitude you could live a healthy, active, successful and long life.

Be critical of yourself. Improve your attitude to life, make time to learn how to live, rather than just concentrating on how to earn a living.

Your destiny depends more on your efforts than you may have realised.

2
WHAT IS THE IMMUNE SYSTEM FOR?

Many things in life are uncertain, but one thing we can be sure of – at some time our living body will die. There are four general reasons for death and each of these is dependent on the immune system.

- The first is injury. In any accident that might occur leaving a body still alive, the main question is 'Can the body be healed?' Although modern medicine does a lot to help, in the long run it is up to the individual body to heal itself.
- The second is infection. Many infectious diseases kill. Many injuries if they are allowed to become infected can kill. We are dependent on an effective immune system that will both recognise foreign materials, such as germs, that enter the body, and reject them.
- The third is non-infectious diseases – degenerative diseases, heart and circulatory diseases, cancer and autoimmune diseases. Many can be caused by either an underactive or overactive immune system.
- The fourth is old age. The age at which we will eventually die naturally will depend on our genes and immune system.

It is important that the immune system remains controlled, organised and competent. It is not a system that we can afford to neglect or confuse. Having an immune system allows us to live in the world, full of potential enemies, and fight back, so ensuring survival of the species.

RECOGNISING SELF AND NON-SELF

We are very sophisticated animals and have very complicated immune systems, but in fact all living things can be attacked by outside influences and have to have some means of recognising 'self' and 'food' and 'enemy'.

Bacteria tend to be thought of as one of the simplest forms of life – they have only one cell – but there are a group of viruses called bacteriophages which infect them and cause them to be 'ill'. Bacteria, therefore, have developed enzymes called endonucleases which can recognise and destroy the attacking viruses' genetic information, thus destroying the viruses. This has to be one of the simplest forms of immunity.

Sponges can distinguish self and non-self. The earthworm, a very simple animal with only about four different types of cell, can make chemicals which either coagulate or burst any foreign invader. The slug, too, has protection from invaders, but its system is not as clever as the higher animals; it is possible to graft part of one slug on to another without the foreign part being rejected.

The simple starfish actually has phagocytic cells. These are specialised cells that live in the body, and can recognise and eat any foreign substance entering it. We have phagocytic cells too and when one reaches the developmental level of the vertebrates, the system becomes very complicated, with even the jawless fish possessing antibodies. Cartilaginous fish such as the dogfish and shark have a spleen and thymus (major immune organs), and the humble frog can suffer from enlarged glands when he is sick.

This concept of self and non-self (or foreign-ness) is fundamental to the understanding and functioning of the immune system, and is dependent, very simply, on the body having a language all of its own, like English or French. Every cell belonging to you has an identity disc or code on its surface, written in amino acids (the building blocks of proteins) instead of letters. We will use letters here so that the principle can be understood.

Take, for example, the following words – t-o-e-s, f-a-c-e, s-t-a-r, b-o-a-t. You can recognise all of these words; they are English and you know what they are. X-y-s-e, d-u-h-p, q-s-n-t, however, are not recognised; these words are rejected.

During the everyday process of living, mistakes are always made. As long as these are spotted early and corrected or eliminated, it does not matter, but if the mistakes are not corrected problems can occur; for example, if the immune system reads b-o-a-t on a cell, it recognises it and does not attack it. If an error occurs to change b-o-a-t to g-o-a-t, any cell with this on will still be recognised and tolerated and the error will not necessarily cause any harm. Should the error alter b-o-a-t to z-o-a-t, then the immune system will not recognise it and will attack as foreign any cells with z-o-a-t marked on their surface.

The thymus gland is the master database computer for the immune system. It lists all codes and informs the various members of the immune army what they can and what they cannot attack. Each group of immune soldiers has its own specific function.

When the body does not recognise self as self, but attacks it as if it were non-self and the situation continues uncorrected, the resulting condition is autoimmune.

IMMUNODEFICIENCY AND IMMUNOSTIMULATION

Because the immune system is so complex and depends on various interactions, it is easy for a variety of defects to occur. They may be genetic, such as the Di George syndrome, where there is an absence of thymus and parathyroid glands, together with other maldevelopments. This condition gives rise to very serious immunodeficiency at birth.

Immunity tends to be weaker during infancy when the immune system is not fully developed, although this is partly compensated for by passive immunity from the mother at birth and by transfer of antibodies in the mother's breastmilk. It is also deficient in old age when the immune system is deteriorating and in cases of malnutrition whether under-, or over- or incomplete-nutrition is the culprit.

Drugs can either intentionally (as in immunosuppression after transplant, etc.) or unintentionally cause immune deficiency, and so can infections; the measles bug suppresses T-cell function, as does the AIDS virus.

Tumours, in particular Hodgkin's disease, myeloma and leukaemias, are associated with immunodeficiency, while polyarthritis and allergies can be associated with B-cell immunodeficiency.

Sometimes, especially in cases of immunodeficiency, the immune system can be stimulated by totally artificial means or by the use of natural mediators like interferons and interleukins. Interferons can be very helpful in the treatment of cancer, especially leukaemia, and is also being tried in AIDS.

Another form of immunostimulation is by transferring antiserum (blood fluid) from people (or originally horses) who have already been exposed to a disease to patients who actively have the disease. This may be a life-saving step, especially in the case of tetanus, hepatitis B or snake bites, as the antibodies in the blood fluid are ready for action right away. Vaccination also stimulates the immune system.

We have an immune system to help us to heal, to keep us healthy and free from disease, to slow down aging and prolong our healthy active life. It is overall an advantage, because all of the successful higher animals have it and we could not normally live without it. We are learning how to manipulate it to further advantage and how to help it. Unfortunately, modern life is also unintentionally discovering how to confuse and disrupt it.

OUR IMMUNE SYSTEM

Advantages
- We are born with a natural resistance to some diseases.
- When stimulated to do so by injury or disease, we have the ability to adapt and so to heal ourselves. This is the adaptive response.
- When faced with an organism – a germ or bug -- that the body does not recognise, the body can usually acquire an immunity to that specific bug, i.e. it can remember it and respond quicker in getting rid of it should it reinfect us again at a later stage in life. This is acquired immunity.
- Vaccination is an artificial way of acquiring acquired immunity. A very small amount of either the dead bug or a specially treated live bug is injected into the body. Because the bug has been killed or treated, it cannot cause disease, but the body's own defences find it, recognise it as foreign, make antibodies to it and remember how to get rid of it. Should you later become infected with the live, active bug, the immune system knows what to do immediately and gets on with it before the bug has a chance to get a hold.

Disadvantages
As with any complicated system, problems occur when the system goes wrong.
- If the system becomes over-active and over-reacts every time there is a stimulus, it causes the problems of hypersensitivity and allergy. Hay fever is a good example. Pollen is relatively harmless and most people tolerate it well, but some people react violently to these tiny particles. The immune system switches on to full red alert as though it was being attacked by a deadly bug. Mast cells (cells involved in allergic responses) burst in their hundreds, histamine is released and the result of all this unnecessary

activity is that fluid pours from the eyes and nose to try to wash away this harmless invader.

- Another problem with having an immune system like ours is that it is programmed to reject everything that is foreign, and that includes transplants. Although the immune system is only doing its job, it poses a problem when it rejects a new kidney, heart, etc. In order to overcome this problem, drugs have to be given to suppress the immune system after the transplant, in the hope of preventing this rejection.

- Autoimmunity is where a body's immune system goes wrong and attacks the body. For example, people with rheumatoid arthritis make antibodies which attack and destroy one type of their own antibodies known as IgG. However, under normal conditions, the immune system tolerates everything in its own body.

Special modifications

- The woman's immune system is altered considerably whilst she is pregnant in order to allow what are after all foreign sperms, and then a different human being, to live inside her body. This is why women with autoimmune diseases often find the symptoms much better whilst they are pregnant, as the immune system is toned down so that her body does not reject the baby as foreign. Even so there are rare cases where the mother's immune system does attack and reject her baby.

3
DOES THE IMMUNE SYSTEM NEED MORE HELP?

Incidences of heart and circulatory diseases, cancer, autoimmune and immune-related diseases are today rising rapidly. Medical science has conquered many of the nasties of the past by improving hygiene standards, by finding ways of killing the bugs which caused disease, by stimulating the body's own immune system to cope with them faster and better, or even by preventing the disease completely with vaccination.

Now we have the modern nasties, and the causes are more difficult to find. Often there is not just one single cause, but a small group of contributory factors, the effects of which work together to cause the disease. Each disease is like a new jigsaw puzzle. We have a few pieces of information which are known to belong to the puzzle. In the centre of the table is a massive heap of odd pieces which may or may not fit our puzzle, or may even fit several puzzles. It is a mammoth task to try them all. Many pieces are dependent on others at the bottom of the pile and consequently the significance of any piece will not always be appreciated.

BALANCE AND CHANGE

When we are in good health, everything is in balance – not perfect, but steady. Everything is working in harmony with everything else, resulting in a complete and healthy whole.

When we are sick, the balance is lost. The immune system battles conscientiously to restore the balance. If it succeeds, we are well again. If it does not, however, other influences may well take advantage of the upset system and join the battle, so putting the system out of balance in other ways. As long as the immune system stays in control, the battle will eventually be won and order restored.

The human body is marvellously adaptable, but it takes time to change and accept new things. At the moment we are not giving it that time. In the blink of an eye in human history, we have changed our lifestyles, air, food, water, movement and sounds. We have added hundreds of new chemicals to our environment and generally upset the balance of nature, as well as the balance of our own bodies. We have accelerated the aging of many of our lakes by tens of thousands of years, and the erosion of the land.

We may also be accelerating the aging of our own immune systems – the system that is responsible for maintaining our balance, our chance for survival on this planet, and whose strengths and weaknesses, mistakes and problems, we pass on to future generations. Because each of us lives for such a short time in history, many are blind to the effects we are having on ourselves. It is like looking in a mirror every day. Each day we look the same as we did yesterday, but when we look back on photographs taken 10 or 20 years previously, we can see the difference.

Worldwide, we have the problem of waste. What do we do with it? The best answer, of course, would be to break it down or build it up into substances which do no harm, but this is difficult, time consuming and expensive. What we do, in effect, is to try to put it somewhere where no one will notice it.

Our immune systems are forced to do the same thing because they are so overworked. Each day we may add a few new chemicals to our bodies – perhaps a new pill or a food additive (of which there are nearly 4,000 now on the market) or a trace of pesticide (something which, after all, is designed to kill living things). The immune system does not always know what to do with these substances; we do not give it time to figure out what to do with one before we add another unknown, and so on. If the immune system cannot detoxify or eliminate wastes from in the body, it has to store them somewhere. Toxic metals are often tidied away in the brain or bone joints – they just build up, year after year. The liver is a common site for build up of many chemicals, as it is one of our main waste disposal units. Build up may occur for tens of years until it gets big enough to cause problems. Unfortunately, by then, turning green cannot reverse all the damage: we need to think green now to prevent us from turning into rusty robots later.

Ironically, at a time when at least half the nation is watching its weight, we need more of some of the nutrients that could to some degree counteract the effects of this extra pollution and stress.

Eating, however, is not always the answer, as much of our refined or treated food does not contain many of the micronutrients we need; the vitamins, minerals, essential fatty acids and natural accessory food substances are regularly removed, along with the roughage and friendly bacteria. The balance of our food is upset and needs to be restored.

THE ENEMIES

We have many enemies in our modern world, some of which we have control over and others which we do not. What each of us needs is a strong well-ordered immune system, equipped with sufficient weapons to be able to deal with any attack. We also need as few enemies as possible, so the more we can eliminate or make friends with these enemies, the better.

Some enemies need to be tackled on a national or worldwide scale. We can tackle them as well if we all do our part, no matter how small that may appear to be. As John Donne said, back in the 16th century, 'No man is an island, entire of itself. Every man is a piece of the Continent, a part of the Main.' We are all in this together, we can all help to restore the balance of life.

Look at the list below. Which enemies are attacking you? Are they strong or relatively weak? Can you counterbalance any of them? How can you help yourself? How can you help others?

Infections

Bacteria, viruses, fungi, protozoa, parasites and worms are all freely available in our world. There is no way of avoiding them completely while still living a normal life. The answer is to get the balance right. Coming into contact with a disease-causing bug does not automatically give it the right to take over. We constantly live with the fungus that causes thrush, for example, or the bug that causes pneumonia. Most of us have an immune system that keeps these under control, as long as we do not alter the balance. Taking a lot of antibiotics that kill our friendly bacteria will allow the irritant fungus (not affected by the antibiotics) to grow into spaces where the friendly bugs would normally be. The result – thrush. If our immune system has been fighting a serious disease and we are recuperating, the pneumonia bug can seize its opportunity and attack whilst the body defences are low, causing serious pneumonia.

Many diseases, including the common cold, are infections and we should try not to pass these on to others, in particular to the very young, the sick and the elderly. It is a poor friend who has an infection and visits someone in hospital who has just had a baby, or has undergone surgery. Keep your unfriendly bugs to yourself.

Stress
Stress can be good or bad, depending on our attitude to it. If stress is causing depression or distress it needs to be minimised, eliminated or balanced, with time spent doing things that give joy and happiness. The excuse of 'I haven't time' just will not work; stress can be a killer and simply stops time altogether.

If, however, you thrive on stress and love every minute of it, it is probably not doing you any harm, but spare a thought for those working with you, who may not be able to take the same sort of pounding.

Unhappiness
Unhappiness is a great immune system suppressor, but again the destruction it can cause is very dependent on our attitude to it. To dwell on it will increase pain. It is better to balance it with more positive thoughts.

Negative attitudes to life
We all make mistakes. No one is perfect – nowhere near it. So it is not worth living with feelings of self-reproach and failure. Negative attitudes are rarely productive. Everyone goes through negative phases in life, but the faster they are recognised and put back into perspective, the faster we become whole again. Years or even lives can be wasted through dwelling on mistakes and problems. The constant negative mind is a powerful immune suppressant.

Noise
Noise can suppress the immune system. Just as it can make objects like glass vibrate until they shatter, so it can shake us. For short periods it might be possible to grit the teeth and bear it, but constant exposure to noise makes the body try to switch off to it (see Chapter 23).

Some people are more sensitive to noise than others. Ear protectors should be worn when the job warrants it. Constant noise saps energy and adversely affects the immune and circulatory systems.

Time
Pressure of modern-day living revolve around time. The failure of an

alarm clock or watch can totally disrupt a day. We have become so dependent on schedules – we jump from deadline to deadline, pouring out hormones into our systems with each leap. Even holidays seem to be a race to fit in as many things as possible.

When really exhausted and in need of a serious holiday, try a peaceful location; eat only what you want to; and above all leave your watch at home. The immune system, the digestive system and indeed the whole body will really enjoy the break.

Radiation

There is no doubt that radiation attacks our body's defences; for example, it can be used to kill bacteria or to destroy cancer cells. We are all exposed to some measure of radiation from the rocks and from the sun – our bodies have evolved to deal with this.

These days, however, we get increasing amounts of radiation. Because of damage to the ozone layer, we get extra radiation from the sun; hence the increase in skin cancers and other related problems. We must take care of our ozone layer and not let it become full of holes.

We are also subject to radiation in medicine and industry. During periods of exposure it is wise to increase antioxidant nutrients to offer maximum protection (see pages 144 and 147).

Exercise

Our bodies were made to move around, otherwise we would have roots, but too much, too little or not the right sort of exercise can inhibit the immune system.

Most of us err on the side of too little exercise (with the excuse that there is not enough time). However, we are probably all aware that our famed athletes do not necessarily have better health or longer lifespans, and many a fanatic jogger has died from a heart attack. Balance, again, is the key, as discussed in Chapter 22. The right type of exercise is also important. Swimming, for example, is great for the heart and lungs, but does not do a thing for the bones.

Nutrition

Starvation or under-supply of any of the nutrients can seriously depress the immune system, but so can over-supply of any one nutrient or of food in general. Care should be taken that supplements are not used to excess or so as to cause an imbalance.

Anti-nutrients are substances which are taken into the body, often along with food, but which do not play a part in body chemistry.

Often these substances not only have no known use, but cause several deleterious immunological reactions.

Chemicals

Our manipulation and use of chemicals affects the lives of every single one of us, and it plays havoc with our immune systems too. There are so many chemicals attacking us daily – cigarette smoke, whether you are an active or passive smoker; exhaust fumes from cars, from boats, from planes, from trains, etc.; smoke from industrial sources, carrying all sorts of things with it; fertilisers and pesticides; industrial and domestic cleaners; thousands of food additives; medicinal, legal and illegal drugs; and many others. How many sources are you exposed to?

Genetics

You may be tempted to say that it all depends on what you are born with. That is true. There is nothing you can do about changing the genetic flaws you have, but there is something you can do about improving your children's and children's children's chances. For example, it has been shown that a zinc deficiency in a mother can take three generations to correct.

The immune system of the foetus is improved with sufficient zinc, methionine, folic acid, vitamin B12 and choline. When these are not well supplied, the immune system is weaker and the immune organs are smaller.

WHAT CONDITION IS YOUR IMMUNE SYSTEM IN?

Make a list of the enemies attacking you. Next to the list, note whether you could eliminate, reduce exposure to, or counterbalance any of these enemies. Does your immune system seem to be coping well or poorly? Indeed, why is it important that the immune system copes well?

- Because the immune system plays a large part in how you age.
- Because the immune system is your housekeeper. It tidies up, cleans up and disposes of the rubbish.
- Because the immune system is your own personal Ministry of Defence, guarding you from enemy attack, whether it is from bugs, radiation or chemical warfare, with enemies from without or whether the enemies are already within.

The secret of keeping your body at peace is to recognise all of the enemies that may be making war against you; to recognise the early

THE EARLY WARNING SIGNS

What we are looking for are changes in any of the following areas.

Hair	Fall, texture, colour, growth, lubrication (greasy or dry).
Head	Dull ache, foggy, floaty, dizzy; sharp pains; pains with movement or behind eyes, flushing or burning sensations.
Eyes	Yellowed whites, twitching, bloodshot, itchy, scratchy, watery; dull pain when moving from side to side; change in vision; tiredness.
Ears	Noises (inside, not an external sound); bubbly, itching, flaking skin; pain; unreal sounds, e.g. own voice loud, other sounds far away.
Nose	Loss of smell; difficulty breathing; mucus, running, itching, full, sore, sneezing.
Mouth	Ulcers, bad taste, bad breath, bleeding gums, loss of taste, coated tongue, bad teeth, sore tongue; difficulty chewing; lack or excess of saliva.
Neck	Stiffness; pain on movement.
Throat	Swollen or painful glands; itchy, sore; difficulty swallowing.
Digestive tract	Indigestion, gas, burning, pain, bloated, constipation, diarrhoea.
Muscles	Weak, painful, numb, tingling, flabby, tense, easily injured.
Joints	Stiff, weak, swollen, painful.
Nails	Ridged, brittle, white spots, split, blue tinged.
Energy levels	High, low, hyperactive, erratic.
Physical	High, low, of short duration; dependent on food and drink intake or stimulants.
Mental	Poor concentration; poor memory, forgetfulness; lack of interest.
Mood change	Depressed, elated, sad, happy, irritable, frustrated, unstable; on or off food; craving specific foods; hooked on any food or drink.

warning symptoms that this enemy or another is quarrelling with your body; and to take steps to ward off the attack before it gets going.

Our bodies tell us quietly if they are having problems, perhaps with tiredness, irritability or a headache. It is only if we take no notice and do not take evasive action that it starts to complain louder and louder, until it eventually shouts 'War'.

There are far too many subtle changes to be listed, some that I may never have come across but that you know only too well. Use the list in the box on page 21 as a guide to minor symptoms that are warning that all is not well and that action is needed to restore harmony. Add your own. Symptoms may well change at different times in life, or you may have a built-in weak spot (e.g. headaches or skin rash) where internal grumbles always show themselves first.

Do not panic if you have any of these. This is not war, yet, but it is always better to sort out small problems on the way rather than to have them all building up and getting tangled with one another, confusing the whole picture later. Your immune system gives you an early warning, indicating that all is not in balance. It is your Ministry of Defence, guarding against invasion. Listen to it and cooperate with it. Supply it with the nutrients that it needs for its weapons. Keep its enemies few in number. Your life depends on it.

4
WHAT THE IMMUNE SYSTEM IS MADE OF

There is no getting round this chapter – it lies at the core of the book. It contains a lot of words and terms that may be unfamiliar to many people, but I have simplified and explained as far as possible. I have hopefully set the chapter out so that it is easy to look up a word that you might come across later in the book.

The whole of the lymphatic system and its associated organs are sometimes referred to as the reticuloendothelial system, or RES. This is a rather outdated term now, but may appear in older books.

THE LYMPHATIC SYSTEM

Basically, immunological battles can occur anywhere in the body, and can involve all organs and tissues, the blood system, etc. We do have a fixed defence framework within the body, though; this is called the lymphatic system, and is outlined in the diagram overleaf.

The lymphatic system is a network of blind-ending vessels which branches throughout the body and contains a clear fluid called lymph. Unlike the blood system, there is no pump to force the lymph around. Movement of this fluid is instead brought about by muscular contraction; hence exercise is important in preventing a sluggish immune system.

Areas of special importance in the immune system are the thymus gland, the bone marrow, blood, spleen, liver (the Kupfer cells), the pituitary and adrenal glands, tonsils, adenoids, appendix, the intestinal Peyer's patches and the lymph nodes.

The lymph nodes, or lymph glands, lie on the lymphatic vessels and are areas of high immunological activity, favourite battle grounds when war on an invader is underway. As you can see from the diagram, the body is, for defence purposes, divided into six areas. Each area has its own nodes (where much of the fighting takes

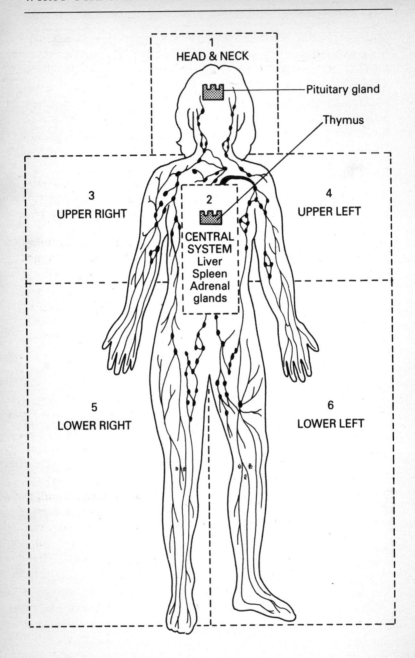

1
HEAD & NECK

Pituitary gland

Thymus

3
UPPER RIGHT

2
CENTRAL
SYSTEM
Liver
Spleen
Adrenal
glands

4
UPPER LEFT

5
LOWER RIGHT

6
LOWER LEFT

The lymphatic system

place); these nodes become the 'enlarged glands' which appear in many infections. Each area tries to confine such immunological battles to within its own boundaries; if, however, an individual's defence is weak, other areas become involved and infected.

The pituitary gland in the brain coordinates all the immune activity in the head and neck area, while the central core (area 2 in the diagram) is the main defence headquarters.

THE THYMUS

This is the master gland of the immune system, situated behind the breastbone in the chest. It is very active before and around the time of birth, but begins to decrease in size and activity from puberty onwards. The growth hormone stimulates it, whilst the sex hormones depress it. It is essential for all T-cell activity (see page 29), and is responsible for distinguishing friend from foe.

Some time before birth the thymus gives all cells an 'identity disc' or code that is recorded in the immune system's memory banks so that the body can recognise its own cells. When cells are coded as self, the body recognises them as self. If an outsider invades the body, the code on it is not recognised and it is attacked as non-self. The system is very complicated and uses amino acids in the same way as we use letters of the alphabet, to build up code 'words'. The average English-speaking person has around 100,000 words available to them: our immune system uses about 10 million.

Thymus activity is closely linked to the rate at which we age. In old age the larger and more active the thymus, the more youthful and resistant we are to disease.

BONE MARROW

The liver of the unborn baby and the bone marrow of the fully developed child and adult provide the stem cells or parent cells from which our blood cells evolve.

At birth and during early childhood, all the bone marrow works flat out to make blood cells. In the adult, though, only the marrow of the central bones are actively producing cells, i.e. the spine, pelvis, ribs and breastbone. This is known as the red marrow. The yellow marrow is much more fatty and is found in the long bones of the arms and legs of the adult. This yellow marrow can be replaced, in some diseased conditions, with red marrow to increase the output of blood cells by up to six times normal levels.

MACROPHAGES AND PHAGOCYTES

Throughout the entire lymphatic system there are cells which are fixed to their posts and not allowed to wander out of their allocated area. These cells are called fixed macrophages and they are programmed to search and sift through whatever passes by them and literally to eat anything which is rubbish or foreign. This process is called phagocytosis, and phagocytes are any cells that feed in this way. This means, in effect, that the whole of our body has guards posted around it whose sole purpose is to look for and get rid of any unwanted material.

Phagocytosis is one of the most primitive forms of feeding, and the method used by many single-celled organisms. The cell recognises food, moves towards it and engulfs it (rather like rolling a piece of dough over and around a small marble), the food eventually ending up inside the cell in a bag or vacuole. Enzymes are then poured on to the food, and it is digested. When a liquid is taken into a cell in the same way, the process is called pinocytosis.

Macrophages and other phagocytic cells in the blood and lymph use this form of feeding to get rid of any of our dead or broken cells and any rubbish or invaders. They get breakfast, lunch, dinner, snacks and midnight feasts, whilst protecting us from attack.

BLOOD AND BLOOD CELLS

The blood is an important part of the defence system. It is made up of a clear yellow fluid, called the plasma, and the blood cells which are suspended in the fluid.

Blood is pumped around the entire body by the heart. Major blood vessels branch into smaller ones and eventually into a network of capillaries so that blood can reach every tissue. It takes oxygen from the lungs to every tissue, and transports the waste carbon dioxide away. It carries food to every tissue and cleans up afterwards by taking waste to the kidneys and liver for eventual removal. It also distributes heat to all parts of the body.

Finally it provides us with a mobile fighting force which is tough enough to seek out and destroy invaders which might harm us, but which is not too proud to empty the body's dustbins daily and to do the general cleaning and tidying necessary to keep us in good working order. Its surveillance goes on 24 hours a day, every day of life, without holidays. This force consists of the white blood cells which are our main immune soldiers; when in good working order, we are able to synthesise around 2,000 new immune cells every second. That's some fighting force, and would be quite a deterrent if germs had any brains.

However, before looking at the various white cells in detail, let's look at some of the other constituents of the bloodstream.

Platelets

Platelets or thrombocytes are small fragments in the blood that are important for our defence because they can get stuck together and coagulate the blood when there is an injury, so preventing all 5 litres pouring out of the hole and leaving the body empty. The plasma contains a substance called fibrin which forms a mesh at the site of the wound, to which the platelets stick. There are between 150,000 and 400,000 platelets per cubic millimetre of blood.

Red blood cells

The red blood cells or erythrocytes are the most common little robots in the blood. There are some 25 million million of them in the body of an adult man, or about 5 million per cubic millimetre. I call these cells robots rather than soldiers because, two or three days before they mature and leave the bone marrow where they are formed, they squeeze out their nuclei; this removes their ability to divide again to form new cells, and they are therefore destined for destruction about four months later.

After leaving the bone marrow they enter the bloodstream, where their role is really only to act as a receptacle for carrying oxygen around the body. They do, however, have suction pads or docking points on their surface. Should any of the 25 million million of them come across something alien whilst on their oxygen delivery rounds, they can arrest it and deliver it to a more senior member of the immune army for sentencing and despatch.

WHITE BLOOD CELLS

The white blood cells or leucocytes are present in the lymph as well as in the blood. Some can even squeeze into tissues when it is necessary to fight an infection. There are fewer of these than there are red blood cells, a mere 25,000 million per average man, or about 8,000 per cubic millimetre.

Just as a country divides its forces into army, navy, airforce etc., so the immune Ministry of Defence divides up its forces, depending on availability of weapons, information and abilities. This is a tricky bit, because they are divided and further subdivided, perhaps a bit like ranks within a particular service.

Granulocytes

Granulocytes are further divided into:

- Polymorphonuclear neutrophils (PMNs for short).
- Eosinophils.
- Basophils.

These cells are all produced from stem cells in the marrow of the flat central bones such as the ribs.

The eosinophils and basophils make up at most 6 per cent of the total white blood cell count and are significant in allergies and worm infections. Along with mast cells in our tissues, they activate an early warning radar system, causing inflammation and drawing attention to the fact that all is not right in that area. Polymorphs and macrophages then rush to their aid in response to the inflammation signals.

Polymorphonuclear neutrophils (PMNs or polymorphs for short) are very small cells with multilobed nuclei, and make up 50 to 70 per cent of the total white cell count. They are phagocytic, gobbling up the foreign bacteria that they come across.

They have a single aim in life, reminiscent of Dr Who's Daleks – 'I will exterminate'. Their determination to carry out their seek, recognise and destroy mission is almost invariably suicidal and they rarely live to fight a second battle. Provided they are not involved in a battle, though, their normal life span is two or three days.

Inside the polymorphs there are little sealed bags called lysosomes which are broken when extermination is needed. Enzymes released from these bleach the alien to death, but are also strong enough to digest the little PMNs as well. Pus found at the site of an infection is a mixture of dead bacteria and the dead PMN army that fought so hard to conquer the enemy.

Monocytes and macrophages

Monocytes are much larger than red blood cells and polymorphs. They are also produced in the bone marrow and then enter the circulation. However they are flexible enough to be able to leave the circulation system through the vessel walls and enter the tissues when needed. When they were found in the tissues they were called macrophages, and it was quite a while before it was realised that the monocytes in the blood were really the same as the macrophages in the tissues (both fixed and wandering).

Although less than 10 per cent of the total white blood cell count consists of macrophages, they are very important. They destroy invaders by phagocytosis and by cleaning our blood, tissues and lymph like efficient selective vacuum cleaners. They are also major chemical factories, capable of making at least 40 different enzymes and immune proteins needed as weapons for the destruction of enemies. Their peacetime chemical activities include making enzymes necessary for clotting of the blood and fat transport.

They are not necessarily killed during an attack and they may live for some time, but even in death they are useful as they are broken down, cannibal-style, by other macrophages and then used as food.

Lymphocytes

Lymphocytes make up somewhere between 20 and 30 per cent of the total white cell count (depending on the degree of infection of the person at a given time). They are the most competent and versatile group for getting rid of unwanted guests. There are around a million million (i.e. 10^{12}) lymphocytes in the average adult body and the principal centres for their production are the lymph nodes, spleen, thymus, Peyer's patches, appendix and other lymphoid tissue; 80 per cent of these cells survive 100 to 200 days.

Lymphocytes have a memory system, so that when second or third invasions by the same kind of bug occur, the immune system can move into action right away instead of wasting time relearning old lessons. Because a reinfection can be tackled right away, it is usually much milder than an initial attack. Lymphocytes have a special method of rapid cell division when under attack, so that they can produce reinforcements almost immediately and you hardly know that you have been into battle. This rapid division is very nutrient dependent; for example, vitamin C levels are crucial. All lymphocytes can move around between tissues, lymph or the bloodstream; none remain fixed, and so a bodywide distribution and memory are ensured.

There are two major types of lymphocytes:
- T cells.
- B cells.

T lymphocytes

Not all T lymphocytes are the same. There are different jobs done by different groups, but all of the T cells have passed through the thymus (the master immune computer) for programming before they are let loose on the body. Some are unarmed and cruise around on surveillance duty, whilst others carry deadly warheads. They provide the initial response to viruses and tumour cells and the rejection of transplants. It takes three to four days after recognition for the T cells to get their act together and attack.

- T helper cells (known as T_H or T_4 cells) help other members of the immune army, but are not armed themselves. They are the body's safeguard against mistakes. If there is a possible invader of questionable identity, it is these T helper cells which determine their fate. These helper cells are also responsible for verifying an invasion and switching the immune system on. The AIDS virus likes to invade these cells, so the victim ends up with few of these helper cells and more suppressor cells (see below). This (much simplified) loss tricks the body into leaving the immune system switched off, even though there is a major invasion taking place.

- T suppressor cells (also known as T_S or T_8 cells) switch off the immune system (both B and T cells) when an infection has passed and recovery is complete. Like the helper cells, the T suppressor cells are not armed.

- Cytotoxic T cells come complete with destructive powers. Their special duty is to search out viruses, etc., which have hidden themselves inside your cells. Most of the body's immune army, when they come across a self cell, recognise it and leave it alone, but the cytotoxic T cell has the ability to seek out and destroy any of the body cells that have a traitor within. They have very strong enzyme 'missiles' which break up and destroy the infected cell. Although they do have a specific target, there is bound to be some damage caused to surrounding cells by the use of such strong weapons.

- Lymphokine-producing T cells also have missiles, but these are aimed at invaders which move in between the body's own cells. Both these and the cytotoxic cells stimulate an increase in activity of the macrophages, as the lymphokines and other chemical weapons do cause a lot of destruction when they have to be used and there are a lot of dead bodies and debris to be cleared away by the normal phagocytic method.

B lymphocytes

B lymphocytes deal mainly with bacteria and with reinfections by viruses that have been encountered before. Attack by a B cell is thus very specific; furthermore, it often requires help from other immune cells.

The task of a B cell is to take any invading bug into the tissues, and there to ascertain its exact size and shape. It then tailor-makes a straightjacket, called an antibody, that will fit that bug and no other. Finally it gets a factory-style production line going which manufactures thousands more of these antibodies which are released back into the body. These, in turn, attach to the bacteria which triggered the reaction in the first place. They search out their targets and attach to them like mini guided missiles. The invader becomes harmless and is held until macrophages or PMNs come along to devour it.

ANTIBODIES

Each antibody is a Y-shaped protein with a clamp or straightjacket on each of the top two arms. Although they are made *en masse* in one of five basic patterns, the end product is tailored specifically to one bug only. The pattern for these receptors is held in memory banks, so that they can be made to order immediately should reinfection occur. This, of course, is the principle upon which vaccination is based, where small quantities of a killed or altered bug are injected into the bloodstream so that antibodies can be made to it; on subsequent infection by the bug that causes the disease, the body can act right away and kill it before it has a chance to get a hold and reproduce. Certain common childhood diseases give a similar response; we get our first taste of them as children and build up an immunity so that we hardly notice subsequent infections. It is, for example, relatively uncommon for an adult to get such complaints as measles and chickenpox if they have had them during childhood; however, it can happen when the immune system is low and not coping effectively.

When first infected, it can take five days for an antibody response. Peak levels of antibodies are then recorded around 14 days. However on reinfection, antibodies can often be detected within 48 hours, and they persist much longer.

Antibodies are often referred to as immunoglobulins. Each molecule of immunoglobulin is made up of two identical light chains (around 200 amino acids each) and two identical heavy chains (which are twice as long). Heavy chains are linked together by what are known as disulphide bonds. This is very significant as some chemicals alter or break disulphide bonds; fluoride is a good example of such a chemical – immunoglobulins are very susceptible to this type of poison.

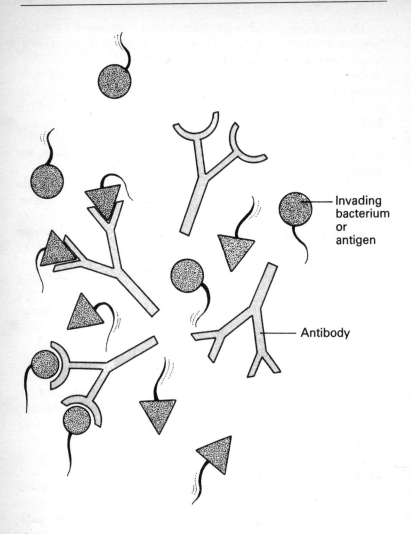

Invading
bacterium
or
antigen

Antibody

Antibodies taking up foreign invaders, such as germs

These immunoglobulins or antibodies are produced by the B lymphocytes in response to infection. The infecting agents or antigens are presented to the B lymphocytes by the T lymphocytes, and these B cells then mature and produce one of five antibody patterns – IgG, IgA, IgM, IgD and IgE.

IgG

This is the most abundant antibody, forming 75 per cent of the total serum immunoglobulin level. It is produced by B lymphocytes, but these in turn require the help of T lymphocytes.

PMNs and macrophages have receptor sites for the tail part of the IgG antibody and so can attach and eat the antibody and its captives when it is ready.

IgG is required by cells which are active in destroying cancer cells, although, unfortunately, they are also involved in transplant rejection and autoimmune diseases.

IgG is actively transported across the placenta and gives both the foetus and the newborn baby (up to six months) protection. The infant usually starts making his own IgG around three months, which is when immunisation programmes often begin.

IgG can activate the complement system (see page 34).

IgA

This type of antibody is found in serum and mucus secretions of the respiratory, genito-urinary and intestinal tracts, where exposure to foreign substances is common. Being protein, immunoglobulins are liable to be digested by the gut enzymes, but IgA can produce a 'secretory piece' which gives it some protection against this. In gastric juices, 80 per cent of the immunoglobulins are IgA.

IgA is often low in those who often suffer with respiratory and gastro-intestinal infections.

IgA's memory and specificity is poor in comparison with the other antibodies, but this is necessary, particularly in the gut, otherwise you could become irrevocably sensitised to almost anything you eat – a boiled egg, for example. People who suffer from food allergy problems probably have malfunctioning IgA; they become over sensitive to certain foods which, in any other person, would not be harmful. Hayfever sufferers are similar; pollen is not really harmful, but some people have a violent reaction to these usually harmless particles.

IgM

IgM is the largest and most primitive immunoglobulin. Its size makes it useful for picking up lots of small antigens, which it can manage ten at a time.

A newborn baby has to synthesise its own IgM as the molecule is too big to cross the placenta. If he does this poorly and the level is too low, the baby could suffer from septicaemia. In contrast, high blood levels of IgM in the newborn indicate that there has been an intra-uterine infection like syphilis, rubella or toxoplasmosis, against which the infant is or has been trying to protect herself/himself.

IgD

Not a lot is known about IgD, but levels are high in the disease of malnutrition, kwashiorkor.

IgE

IgE is attracted to mast cells (cells involved in allergic responses) and basophils. It is associated with all forms of allergy including hayfever, asthma, hives, itching, rhinitis, etc. People who suffer from allergies usually make too much IgE, and an allergic tendency can be passed on to children, although the allergy may not take on the same symptoms and form.

SERUM PROTEINS

The serum is that part of the blood which is not the cells. The proteins in it (which include the immunoglobulins) are very important in immunological reactions.

Interferons are special proteins produced against viruses, and they are sometimes released into the serum. Many of the other serum proteins are used to maintain water balance or as part of cell nutrition.

The complement proteins are a group of serum proteins which circulate in the blood. When an invader bumps into and stimulates one of them (called a C_3 protein) it alters chemically and attracts other complement proteins to it. When four to six complement proteins are joined together in a special order, the jigsaw is complete and the invader is killed and phagocytosed. There are two ways to fit the pieces together; one is known as the classical way, the other the alternative route. The jigsaw pieces stay separate in the blood most of the time and are only fitted together in the correct order when the destructive weapons need to be released; this prevents continuous

firing of weapons which, in the absence of an enemy, would destroy
your own cells.

THE WEAPONS OF THE IMMUNE SYSTEM

The whole body is our battleground; some parts of the immune
army will move to almost any site necessary in order to destroy
invaders. However, the main sites for the recruitment of
immune soldiers is in the foetal liver, bone marrow and
lymphoid organs. Officers in the T service then go through a
final programming in the thymus. Immune soldiers, when
ready, are sent out into the blood and lymphatic systems for
surveillance duty and real action.

- Red blood cells merely arrest invaders and pass the
  package to the white blood cells to deal with.

There are several types of white blood cells.

- Macrophages and polymorphs eat the enemy. Macrophages make enzymes needed for weapons of war and
  peaceful activities, and they also take on the housekeeping
  role.
- Eosinophils and basophils cause inflammation and warn of
  attack.
- B lymphocytes are ordered to attack only specific targets.
  They need one to two weeks to make a good supply of antibody and to remember their targets so that they can supply
  antibody faster should there be a second attack.
- T lymphocytes regulate the immune system and decide
  whether it goes into battle or withdraws. Some of its officers attack specific invaders, either in or between cells.
- There are various serum proteins, like complement and
  immunoglobulins, and also other substances like interferons and lysozymes which can be mobilised for attack
  when needed, these usually travel around the body,
  disarmed as it were, until needed.

Finally, let's look at two terms that often cause confusion:

- Antigens are anything which provokes an antibody response.
  Bugs which cause disease are said to be antigenic because their
  presence in the body causes the B cells to make antibodies to
  coat and help destroy them.
- Antibiotics are a sort of mercenary chemical force which is

sometimes sent in by doctors to help combat a bacterial infection. Antibiotics are not made in the body, and should not be confused with antibodies – they are not the same thing at all.

5
HOW THE
IMMUNE SYSTEM
WORKS

Next, we need to understand how the immune system works, the battle tactics used and which units are called into play at any time. It is also useful to know how to help, or at least not to hinder, our own private army.

Immunity literally means being exempt from getting something again. The study of immunology is the study of how the body, surrounded by an increasingly polluted environment, defends itself; it is the study of life from before birth, through the hazards of living, to inevitable death.

DEFENCES AGAINST EXTERNAL THREATS

The immune system has to be able to destroy anything which threatens the body – the winner gets life, the loser death.

Adaptations for certain exceptions

It is no good destroying everything that is foreign that enters the body. We need food, for example, to live, but it is foreign, non-self; the gut therefore has to have its immune system adapted so that we can take foreign material into it. We can usually eat an egg with no ill effects, but the egg could not be injected straight into the bloodstream – the immune system there would attack it immediately.

In order for us to reproduce, foreign sperm has to enter the female body. The sperm, which is non-self, therefore has to come complete with local immune suppressors so that it can survive. The pregnant woman's whole immune system has to change a lot in order to allow a completely different body to live inside her for nine months.

Many bacteria are unfriendly, but not all of them; some are necessary for our normal everyday existence, and it is very important that our immune system does not attack them. When our friendly gut bugs are destroyed with antibiotics, we are left open to attack by fungi and other pathogens (harmful organisms). We need our friendly neighbourhood bugs in the gut, on the skin, in the genito-urinary tract and other mucous membranes so that foreigners cannot establish themselves and change the environment to our disadvantage.

At a more fundamental level, civil war within the body must be avoided – the immune system must not attack its own men (a difficult task when there are several million million of them). It is also important that weapons intended for use on invaders do not accidentally destroy our own defenders; they need to be carefully stored and disarmed for day-to-day living.

NON-SPECIFIC IMMUNITY

There are two systems of immunity working side by side. One is specific immunity, where the body concentrates on dealing with a specific situation, say chickenpox or pregnancy. The other is a very general immunity which could be used for lots of problems. We will deal with the non-specific or general immunity first.

Immunity due to species

Have you ever seen a dog with a cold or the measles? Probably not, because the germs that cause these diseases do not affect the dog. The rabies virus, however, will attack both man and dog once it can get inside our or the dog's skin; the rabies virus cannot penetrate healthy skin, so usually this disease is only transmissible through a bite or wound.

The rat is not susceptible to the diphtheria bacteria and can live quite happily in a sewer, whilst man and guinea-pig are highly susceptible to the disease and would not survive long in such an environment. The myxomatosis virus favours rabbit, whilst the bacteria causing leprosy and syphilis prefer man. By virtue of being human, we can safely say that we do not suffer from fowlpox or potato blight.

We are thus not susceptible to all disease-causing organisms.

Immunity due to genetics

There are some illnesses which are genetically determined. Most of us, for example, do not suffer from haemophilia. It is not an infection; you cannot catch it; you cannot make it go away by altering diet or exercise. It is genetically determined who has it and who does not.

Biochemical barriers to infection

We have many chemicals inside us which destroy unwanted bugs and other substances. Their effect is general, not specific to any one kind of bug.

Lysozyme

Blood, eye fluids and many of our cells carry an enzyme called lysozyme which is just such a chemical. It is sometimes called the natural antibiotic, as it destroys bacteria. Fleming discovered both lysozyme and penicillin. Lysozyme is found in dilute solution in body fluids. In the immune cells, however, it is concentrated in special little packets called lysosomes. When these burst, this concentrated lysozyme is released and kills the invading bacteria. It will, of course, destroy some of the body cells as well, so it is important that these packets of concentrated lysozyme remain intact and only get broken when there are disease-causing bacteria to attack.

Interferon

Interferon is an antiviral agent, but again it is non-specific, i.e. it will act against any virus that it finds lurking about. It prevents a virus from multiplying inside the cell, probably by closing down the power source of that cell, and it can also prevent neighbouring cells from being infected.

Most tissue cells can secrete interferon when infected, as long as they have sufficient vitamin C and manganese. Sometimes cells become diseased and altered (e.g. cancer cells); these may lose their ability to produce interferon and so are relatively easily invaded by other viruses. This is why it is difficult to pinpoint cancer-causing viruses; it is a chicken and egg situation – did the virus cause the cancer or did it move in afterwards?

The ability to make interferon is coded in our genes, our inherited material. Indeed the human interferon gene can now be synthesised; it is a very large gene of over 500 units or nucleotides, but when it is inserted into the bacterium called *E. coli*, the bacterium will make large quantities of interferon. This could obviously be very useful in medicine, although it is not the whole of the answer to the elimination of harmful viruses.

Complement

The complement system is also non-specific. It comprises a group of proteins which come together, when stimulated, to bring about the destruction of unwanted material. Complement also attracts PMNs that clear up after battle, and seems to instigate the inflammatory process.

One method of complement fixation is dependent on calcium, the other on magnesium, but either method of activation is a valuable help to other parts of the immune system. Tumour cells, for example, can often survive in the presence of antibody alone, but the addition of complement causes their cell membranes to become fragile and patchy and then for the cells to die. In particular, complement proteins have been shown to be able to neutralise the herpes simplex virus.

As we saw in the previous chapter, in order to prevent their uncontrolled attack the complement proteins are usually found separated in the blood. It is only when they come together in the correct order, stimulated by a threatening situation, that they cause destruction. It is rather like taking a gun apart and only putting it together when there is something to shoot; it prevents it going off by accident. We also have an inhibitor, the safety catch, which stops the action after the battle has passed. In exceptional cases there may be a deficiency of the inhibitor, and this condition is described as hereditary angioneurotic oedema. Complement deficiencies are rare, but a few hereditary deficiencies can cause recurrent infections and renal disease. Nutritional deficiencies of calcium or magnesium may also inhibit its action.

Other chemicals

Blood, sweat, tears and tissue fluids have various other biochemically active anti-bug substances, such as properdin, beta-lysins, basic proteins (such as protamine and histone), basic peptides (such as leukins and phagocytins) and basic polyamines (such as spermine and spermidine). It is sufficient for general knowledge just to know that such chemicals exist in the body.

Finally, the acidity of our skin and stomach secretions is a barrier to infection, as are sufficient zinc levels in seminal and amniotic fluid. Bile salts and essential fatty acids in the intestines also deter pathogens.

Physical barriers to infection

We also have physical barriers that protect us from attack. Primarily, the skin keeps us in and, to a degree, separate from the rest of the world. Secretions from its glands contain antifungal and antibacterial substances to protect the outer horny layer from attack. We also have many friendly bacteria on the skin surface that prevent invasion by less friendly ones. As long as our skin is intact, we are relatively safe from the bugs which surround us; however, if the skin has wounds, there is always the risk of infection.

Obviously, to enable us to breathe, eat, excrete and reproduce, we have to have entrances to our bodies. These, in turn, have special skin surfaces and secretions to protect them. The damp, mucous membranes of the nose and respiratory tract, for example, along with the hairs and cilia (microscopic hairs), trap many would-be invaders. Some well known respiratory bugs, like the ones causing influenza, interfere with the sweeping action of the cilia, which is why they are so successful.

There are no cilia in the gut, but mucus and peristalsis (the constant pushing movement of the gut) prevent much bacterial growth; the churning action and acidity of the stomach also prevent infection. Infection occurs when the mucous membrane is damaged or when peristalsis slows down (as in constipation), but can also be caused by food poisoning.

Tissues and cell walls, as well as the blood-brain barrier and placental barrier, all prevent free exchange of material and so, to a degree, protect us from some things that might harm us. Coughing, sneezing and crying also get rid of potentially harmful substances. Ways of improving our physical barriers will be dealt with in Chapter 6.

Temperature

Many of the bugs that cause us to be ill are very fussy about the central heating system; for example, the bacillus that causes TB in humans will not infect cold-blooded animals. Hens do not usually contract anthrax, but if their temperature is lowered they can be infected. Bugs which cause gonorrhoea are killed above 40°C; before antibiotics became available, raising the body temperature was a common treatment for this condition.

Macrophages and other immune cells work better at a temperature above normal body temperature; this is why fever often accompanies infection. If we try to lower a fever, (providing it is not life threatening) we could be putting our immune cells at a disadvantage – mild fever aids the immune response. Obviously a very high temperature, over which the body appears to have lost control, must be lowered or it could be dangerous in itself.

SPECIFIC IMMUNITY

Specific immunity is where the immune system is specialised to act against a particular bug or condition. It is usually divided into active and passive immunity and both are further divided into natural and artificial immunity.

Passive immunity

This is where antibody cells or antitoxins are transferred from an immune person to a non-immune person. This happens naturally when immunity is passed from mother to child via the placenta or in colostrum (a baby receives colostrum whilst breastfeeding). Artificially, it may be used in medicine to treat tetanus, snake bite or those with immune deficient diseases.

All passive immunity is of short duration. Once the substance passed on to the non-immune person is used up, the beneficial effects are lost.

Active immunity

This is when the body's own immune cells recognise a specific bug or substance and react to it. It has a memory, to recognise and deal with the problem on subsequent occasions. So B and T cell activity, as well as some macrophage activity, is specific.

Natural active immunity occurs during infection, and artificial active immunity happens when we are immunised.

SUMMARY

In this and the previous chapter you have read about the organs, cells and other components of the immune system:
- Blood system.
- Lymphatic system.
- Lymph nodes.
- Thymus gland.
- Pituitary gland.
- Liver.
- Spleen.
- Adrenal glands.
- Peyer's patches in the gut.
- Appendix.
- Tonsils and adenoids.
- Skin.

- Red blood cells.
- Platelets.
- White blood cells or leucocytes, consisting of the macrophages, granulocytes (PMNs, eosinophils and basophils) and lymphocytes (T and B cells).
- Antibodies.
- Complement proteins.
- Various other antibacterial and antiviral chemicals, especially interferon and lysozyme.

You have also found out what enemies your immune system is up against, from the obvious attackers like bacteria, viruses, fungi, protozoa and worms, through radiation, pollution, fumes, smoke, fertilisers, pesticides, drugs, industrial and domestic chemicals, food additives, to accidental damage.

It will also become apparent in later chapters that too much food, or lack of nutrients, as well as stress, inappropriate exercise and genetics all have important roles in how we can use the marvellous immune system effectively.

In the accompanying diagrams I have tried to sum up the usual action of the body when attacked. It is, of necessity, very general and involves first humoral immunity in the first five lines of defence, then cell mediated immunity. Use the diagram on pages 44 and 45 alongside the following numbered paragraphs.

1 Firstly, the surface barriers of the body have to be broken in some way to allow entry of a germ. If these barriers are kept in good condition and intact, infections and hence illness are less likely. The main physical barriers are skin, gut lining and membranes of the respiratory and genito-urinary tract. Sometimes one of these physical barriers will fail.

2 Naturally occurring antibiotics such as lysozyme are the next defence to be encountered.

3 Phagocytic cells are also in the body fluids, ready to attack. Should these first three defences fail, the next defence mechanisms are available.

4 Complement proteins will either act alone to break open the germ (and hence destroy it via the alternative pathway), or they will act with a phagocyte to destroy it.

5 If natural antibiotics, phagocytes and the alternative complement pathway are not entirely successful, the B lymphocytes will have been making antibodies which are eventually released. These may also be used with complement proteins in the classical pathway to destroy germs.

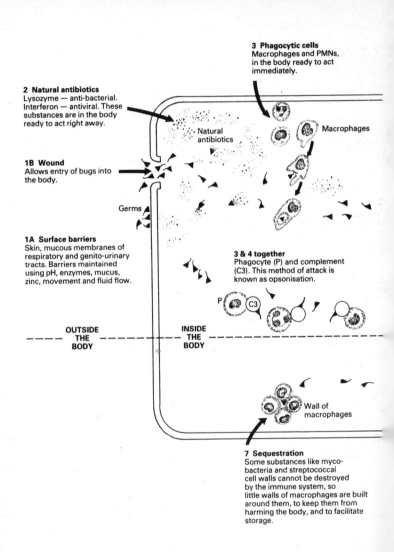

3 Phagocytic cells
Macrophages and PMNs, in the body ready to act immediately.

2 Natural antibiotics
Lysozyme — anti-bacterial. Interferon — antiviral. These substances are in the body ready to act right away.

Macrophages

Natural antibiotics

1B Wound
Allows entry of bugs into the body.

Germs

1A Surface barriers
Skin, mucous membranes of respiratory and genito-urinary tracts. Barriers maintained using pH, enzymes, mucus, zinc, movement and fluid flow.

3 & 4 together
Phagocyte (P) and complement (C3). This method of attack is known as opsonisation.

P   C3

OUTSIDE THE BODY

INSIDE THE BODY

Wall of macrophages

7 Sequestration
Some substances like myco-bacteria and streptococcal cell walls cannot be destroyed by the immune system, so little walls of macrophages are built around them, to keep them from harming the body, and to facilitate storage.

Humoral immunity and cell-mediated immunity

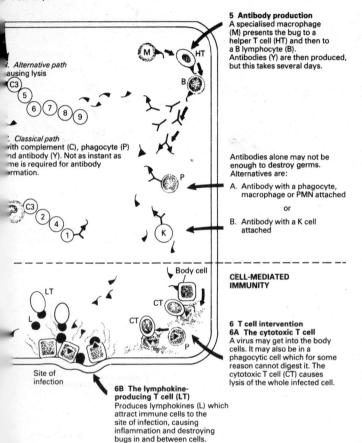

Complement
A Opsonisation
B Alternative path
C Classical path

5 Antibody production
A specialised macrophage
(M) presents the bug to a
helper T cell (HT) and then to
a B lymphocyte (B).
Antibodies (Y) are then produced,
but this takes several days.

Alternative path
ausing lysis

Classical path
with complement (C), phagocyte (P)
nd antibody (Y). Not as instant as
me is required for antibody
rmation.

Antibodies alone may not be
enough to destroy germs.
Alternatives are:

A. Antibody with a phagocyte,
     macrophage or PMN attached

or

B. Antibody with a K cell
     attached

Body cell

**CELL-MEDIATED
IMMUNITY**

**6 T cell intervention
6A The cytotoxic T cell**
A virus may get into the body
cells. It may also be in a
phagocytic cell which for some
reason cannot digest it. The
cytotoxic T cell (CT) causes
lysis of the whole infected cell.

Site of
infection

**6B The lymphokine-
producing T cell (LT)**
Produces lymphokines (L) which
attract immune cells to the
site of infection, causing
inflammation and destroying
bugs in and between cells.

6   Finally, special T cells recognise the invaders that got away and are hiding in between the cells, whilst others recognise cells which have been infected and get rid of them.

7   Most dead bodies and rubbish are eliminated, but sequestration is a final resort for stuff which cannot be dealt with any other way. This involves building macrophage walls around the offending material.

NUTRITIONAL SUPPORT

Natural antibiotic production, production of complement proteins, ability to carry out phagocytosis and to digest the prey are dependent on vitamin C, so it is easy to see why an increased consumption of this vitamin at the time of infection (rather than at the time of symptoms) is crucial. The vitamin C at the time of infection immediately increases the instant protection: taken a day or so later, it will be far less effective.

Complement production is calcium and magnesium dependent, whilst interferon production is manganese dependent. Calcium is also needed for fever production which aids our immune soldiers. All three nutrients are commonly deficient in the refined diet, although we are getting much more conscious about calcium these days.

We have seven main ways of defending ourselves. As we have just seen, methods two, three and four are all impaired by something as simple as vitamin C deficiency. The effect of nutrition on the immune system will be dealt with in detail in Chapters 13 to 17, and other things which affect it will be dealt with in Chapters 18 to 21.

The next chapter deals with the first step, how we can improve our physical barriers to make them less prone to attack.

6
IMPROVING YOUR PHYSICAL BARRIERS

Imagine that you have just bought a castle. It is where it is; you cannot pick it up and move it to another location. Similarly, you cannot knock it down and build it in a different shape; you are stuck with the basic structure and its location.

Your body is your castle, and likewise you are stuck with a few unchangeables. You have to make the best of the genes that you have and the species that you are, but you can do a lot to improve the physical structure, to make it look better, last longer and wear better. There are lots of improvements you can carry out which will make it more resistant to attack, better able to be defended and less likely to turn on itself.

Any germ (I use the words germ or bug as very general terms, covering any infecting organism whether it be bacteria, virus, fungus, protozoa or whatever) has to gain entry into the body. We know how our physical barriers try to prevent this, but how can we help? How do we hinder?

THE SKIN

The skin probably takes the most abuse. It is obviously our main barrier to the rest of the world. It is a living organ which needs feeding and cleaning, like any other living thing. It also needs to breathe. If we painted our skin all over, we would die.

To make its cell walls strong and resistant to attack, the skin needs plenty of vitamin A or its precursor, beta-carotene. It needs plenty of zinc in order to fight bacteria, protein and vitamin C for collagen repair, vitamin E and essential fatty acids to slow the weathering and aging processes, and, most of all, it needs to maintain its acid balance. Yet most people wash several times daily with plenty of soap and water.

Sweat and soap

Every schoolboy knows that frequent washing with soap is wrong, but he will probably grow up conditioned to its use and may even shave and merely wipe the soap off. Most soap is alkaline and, whilst it is great for removing dirt, it makes the skin more susceptible to infection if it is not rinsed off properly. Soap also harms our commensals, the helpful bacteria living on the skin that prevent its occupation by less desirable bugs. These commensals make a living by eating up our old skin cells, our unwanted secretions and day-to-day dirt. They do not mind water, but they split when faced with soap.

The sebaceous secretions and sweat of the skin contain bactericidal and fungicidal (-cidal meaning to kill) fatty acids, triglycerides and wax alcohols. The sweat gland secretions, for example, contain lactic acid, amino acids, uric acid and ammonia and are normally at an acid pH of around 5.5. Soap solution is higher than pH 7 (which is neutral), this higher figure indicating alkaline conditions. (The higher the pH figure, the more alkaline the conditions; the lower the figure, the more acid the conditions.)

Although most people have little respect for sweat, the real healthy stuff that gives you your true body odour can be a powerful attractor to the opposite sex. However, the unhealthy, rancid zinc-deficient alkaline version that people try to wash away or spray over these days most definitely has the opposite effect, and encourages rather than discourages the growth of less desirable bugs.

Feet are positioned as far away from the nose as possible and are notorious for their pungent sweaty smell. Yet in reality, the soles of the feet (and the hands) are deficient in sweat and sebaceous glands, and hence in antimicrobial secretions, which is why they are always more susceptible to infections like athletes' foot and verrucas, as well as warts. These areas are sometimes referred to as alkaline gaps. Feet do not smell to annoy you. It is a cry for help, a warning that all is not right, that conditions are too alkaline, too wet, not ventilated enough, zinc deficient or whatever. Happy feet do not have to smell.

Talc

The use of talcum powder is an equally strange habit. Why is it used? To make you smell better? To keep the skin dry? As it is usually applied after a bath, you should be smelling your best already. If you dried yourself properly, where is the need to dry with powder? Talc clogs the pores so that our beneficial secretions cannot get out. It flies around and can be breathed in, preventing cilia and mucous membranes from working properly. If it gains entry to the blood through a wound, it is one of the substances that the immune system does not know what to do with and so has to sequestrate. This means that it has to build tiny walls of macrophages around it for the rest of your life to keep it harmless and packaged. Packages often get stored in joints, out of the way. A young person can take a lot of this. However, with age and a lifetime of package storing, the joints get full up, and fed up, and start to complain.

Cosmetics

Many people are sensitive to certain cosmetics; whilst it is important to be able to use some (they can do wonders for self-confidence, as well as for looks), it is equally important to be careful which ones you use. Remember, the skin is a living organ, just like your heart, stomach and liver, and you would not smear cosmetics over those.

Face paints have been used for centuries, but are not always beneficial. Once upon a time lead was used in face powders to lighten the skin; it was absorbed, and many fashionable ladies died of lead poisoning. Aluminium is often used in aftershaves and antiperspirants; it is not a good idea to use these immediately after shaving, when there may be some skin damage. One has to be particularly careful of lipsticks, too – after all, you do eat them. They have to be highly coloured, and many contain aluminium.

The skin may be sensitive to some dyes and chemicals in cosmetics, so always avoid the ones that cause soreness or irritation, even if it means throwing a new purchase away; you can buy a new foundation cream or lipstick, but not a new skin. Choose cosmetics carefully and write to the manufacturers concerning contents. If enough of us ask questions, they will know what sort of product to make and which chemicals to avoid.

Radiation

Midday sun has most of the damaging ultraviolet radiation (early morning and late afternoon sunshine is higher in the less damaging form of UV and so it is a better time to sunbathe). We tend to think of moisturisers as reversing the drying out effect of the sun, but according to one London skin specialist they actually enable the damaging UV to penetrate deeper into the skin, so it is not a good idea to use such products before going into the sun.

You can also help to protect the skin from the sun's attack by eating foods high in para-amino-benzoic acid (PABA) and beta-carotene. Both of these help in the prevention of skin cancer. PABA and pantothenic acid (both B vitamins) are essential for making melanin, which produces that protective tan; it is therefore useful to ensure sufficient quantities in the summer diet. Because we refine out a lot of the B vitamins, PABA is often deficient. Even red- and fair-haired people can get a protective tan by ensuring sufficient PABA. The richest food sources of PABA are liver, eggs, yeast and wheatgerm. The best source of beta-carotene are carrots, apricots and other orange or red fruits and vegetables. Supplements are often advisable during the summer.

Damage to the skin
Damage to the skin is an obvious method of entry for germs.

Bites by snakes and animals always require medical advice, but insect bites are very common and rarely require such help. Most insect stings, including that of the bee, tend to be acid and one teaspoon of sodium bicarbonate to a glass of water is alkaline enough to neutralise and soothe a little. Wasp stings are an exception, and require vinegar.

Insects are deterred by the body odour (detected only by the insect) of a person who has sufficient vitamin B_2; given the choice of a B_2 deficient individual or someone who has sufficient, an insect will choose the deficient one any day. Of course, if there is no choice you will still be fair game, but at least the insect does not enjoy his meal as much! It is worth making sure that you are not B_2 deficient during the insect season if you always seem to be the restaurant of choice.

The malarial bug loves para-amino-benzoic acid (PABA). Anti-malarial treatment is based on removing this B vitamin from the body. Whilst fine, and definitely preferable to getting malaria in the short term, breaks should be given from this treatment in the long term.

Diseases can be spread by insects, and it is definitely worth taking evasive action in other countries where insect bites can be more dangerous, whether by using insect repellants or avoiding exposure during the witching hours of vampire mosquitoes. I well remember, when we moved to the Seychelles, spending the first evening standing barefoot on an isolated tropical beach, gazing at the moon reflected on the water. I even more vividly remember waking the next day and vowing never to do it again as I surveyed and felt the damage caused by the sandflies and mosquitoes which had banqueted on me the night before!

Other methods of puncturing the skin (injections, tatoos, ear piercing, etc.) are not advisable, unless, of course, medically necessary.

Finally, infections can be passed on by touch, especially when food is handled by an infected person. This brings us on to the next area where we can take steps to avoid infection.

THE GUT

Most of the gut is not supplied with temperature sensitive nerves. The mouth does have such nerve endings, though, acting as a safety measure – if it is too hot for the mouth, it is too hot for the stomach. Remember, the stomach can get cooked, just like any other bit of meat, and years of consuming food and drink which is too hot is bound to decrease its effectiveness.

Too much liquid taken with your food will dilute digestive enzymes and stomach acid, both of which kill bugs and digest food. Take most of your fluid intake between meals. However, food poisoning is much more likely to occur when eating raw, undercooked, stale or reheated foods. Deep fried foods like chips are unlikely to cause food poisoning so, if eating out, weigh up the hygiene standards. If in doubt, go for deep fried foods and counterbalance this consumption of fat by cutting down during the following days.

At home, of course, food poisoning can be avoided 99 per cent of the time with good food hygiene, such as washing, covering food which is left to stand in the open, refrigeration, paying attention to sell-by-dates, not keeping food too long, separating raw meats and fish from cooked meat and other produce, etc. But there will always be that odd 1 per cent chance, where food is contaminated at source and you do not know about it – until afterwards.

Fibre

The intestines are coiled tubes through which food is passed. If the diet is sufficient in fibre, the passage of food will be quite speedy and will scour the tubes. But if fibre or water is lacking, or peristalsis (the pushing movement of the muscles of the gut) is inefficient, then food residues can build up on the walls of the intestines. This encourages the growth of undesirable bugs and can cause a lot of problems for the immune system.

Such a build up in the large intestine can lead to constipation, and although this may be relieved temporarily by various pills and potions, the diet and lifestyle needs to be looked at seriously in order to correct the cause. Constipation is a minor symptom, but if not investigated and corrected the problem could turn into something more serious.

To improve the passage of food residues and faeces, it is wise to include more fibre foods in the diet. It is not a good idea, however, to sprinkle wheat bran on to everything; this type of fibre irritates many people's gut, especially those sensitive to wheat, and it also tends to hold on to valuable minerals and prevent them from being absorbed by the body. This dry type of fibre is best taken at one meal, say breakfast, and not sprinkled on foods throughout the day. As with most things, you can overdo it.

Egestion – the removal of faeces from the body – is a method of removing toxins from the body before they can be absorbed, as well as removing unwanted bugs.

THE GENITO-URINARY TRACT

The acidity of urine deters many bugs, but of equal importance in this respect is urine flow; there is much less chance of urinary tract infection if good quantities of fluid are drunk and flushed through the tubes. Any condition which slows or prevents flow will cause urinary tract infections, and this includes not drinking enough. Elderly people often lose their desire to drink; the thirst mechanism seems to decline with age, the body somehow forgets to say that it is thirsty and so the elderly suffer more from this condition. The fluid consumed should have a high water content – water itself, dilute squashes, dilute (not strong) tea or coffee, herb teas, etc. Lemonades, colas, spirits etc., do not improve the condition.

Good zinc levels in seminal and amniotic fluid are essential to deter bugs in these areas. Men lose a lot of zinc with every loss of semen. A high sex drive will therefore probably mean zinc supplementation is advisable in this country, where zinc levels are low anyway – vegetarians are especially vulnerable as a lot of our zinc comes from meat. Women, too, need zinc, especially when they are pregnant. The vagina is obviously very susceptible to infection. Remember when sperm enters the vagina, they come complete with their own immunosuppressants and bugs.

Antibiotic treatments which kill bugs in the genito-urinary tract and gut can often also predispose you to fungal infections like thrush. After a course of antibiotics, it is therefore helpful to take a course of B vitamins and eat yoghourt to encourage the growth of friendly bugs again as quickly as possible. Should an individual be sensitive to milk or its products, lactobacilli supplements are available instead of yoghourt. Lactobacilli in the vagina ferment glycogen and acidify the pH to around 4; when they are not present the pH rises and other pathogenic bugs thrive, causing further problems.

RESPIRATORY TRACT

The bactericidal and viricidal secretions in the mucous membranes of the respiratory tract, as well as the cilia (microscopic hairs that sweep germs and debris out of the respiratory tubes), do a good job. However, we frequently hinder these. Smoking – active or passive – damages the membranes and cilia, as well as drying out the secretions. Pollution, too, lays down deposits and clogs these mechanisms. Toddlers are particularly at risk, either in pushchairs or on foot, as they are often right down at exhaust-pipe level; sitting them higher up on the end of the pram, or walking through less congested back streets, does help, especially if the main street has lots of traffic lights or car jams – there are more emissions from this type of traffic than from free flowing traffic.

Central heating is very drying, and for health as well as economy is best kept on as low a setting as possible. It is also a good idea to keep a bowl of water near a heat source so that the air is not quite so dry. A bowl of flowers will do very well as an alternative if you don't like the look of a bowl of water; they do, of course, die quickly near radiators, but that is because they are living things too and have a similar problem.

Bugs in the air do not usually cause us a problem as the respiratory tract normally deals with these. However, if someone sneezes or coughs near your breathing space, you may get an extra heavy dose of bugs such as flu – there may be too many at any one time to be dealt with. This is why colds and flu are so catching. It is possible to avoid a major attack, however, if you recognize that the person near you is infected. Before any symptoms show – in fact as soon as possible – take a gram of vitamin C and a zinc supplement that can be sucked, and maintain a high level of vitamin C for the next two or three days. The secret is to catch the bug before it catches you, not to wait until you have the symptoms. Dose is also important and varies from individual to individual. For some, 1 gram per day is enough to prevent the infection; others may need 4 to 6, or even 10 grams. People who are already ill will usually need more than those who are perfectly fit. You need to find your level, and it may take a cold or two before you get it right.

Commensal organisms live in the respiratory tract as well as on the skin, in the gut and genito-urinary tracts. Anything which alters the normal flora of these regions is likely to be followed by replacement of them with pathogenic organisms. We therefore need to keep our friendly bugs happy and deter the unfriendly ones from moving in.

7
INFECTIOUS DISEASES

We cannot avoid being infected by bugs at some time or another, but infection by some microorganisms can mean infection for life. A very successful organism will live inside a body without killing its host; however, any alteration in the state of the host's immune system could then give that organism the advantage. We all pick up hitch-hiker bugs on our journey through life; they then just wait for an opportunity to take over in the driving seat. Maintenance of a strong immune system throughout life is vital.

In fact it is really an unsuccessful bug that kills, because it then has to move on and find a new home. However, there are some around and no matter how good our immune system is such bugs will probably manage to wreck it. Pathogenic organisms are not without tricks of their own.

DEALING WITH BACTERIA

Some bacteria try to evade our immune army by forming a protective capsule around themselves; examples are the streptococci that cause sore throats and the bacteria that cause flu, pneumonia and meningitis. Infection by these can cause tissue damage and autoimmunity if the body's immune system or medicine cannot keep them in check. Streptococci, for example, if not controlled can cause acute rheumatism, rheumatic fever or kidney damage. The bug treponema, which causes syphilis, may also initiate autoimmune problems by mimicking the amino acid markers which code for cardiolipin (in heart muscle cells). The immune cells have the choice of ignoring treponema, and allowing the disease to progress, or attacking the treponema along with the cardiolipin-containing heart muscle cells – a no-win situation.

Other bacteria have cell walls which are resistant to digestion by phagocytic enzymes; examples include a food poisoning bug, salmonella, and the bacteria causing TB and leprosy.

Then there are the bacteria that produce chemicals that attack the immune system in an attempt to immobilise it. Examples include tetanus, diphtheria, cholera, dysentery, abscesses (staphylococci), scarlet fever and botulism. The toxins these bacteria produce can obviously continue to cause tissue damage, even if the bacteria are killed.

Bacteria like pseudomonas, listeria and *E. coli* only cause problems when the immune system is not sufficient for some reason, for example because of immaturity, pregnancy, illness or old age.

But not all bacteria have these special talents, and most of them can be dealt with very effectively by a competent immune system.

DEALING WITH VIRUSES

Viruses are very difficult to study as they are so small and not easy to detect. Many have been implicated in cancers, like the hepatitis B and the glandular fever viruses, but it is difficult to know whether they cause the cancer or just move in after the cancer has become established.

Viruses do not have protective cell walls. Furthermore they cannot reproduce by themselves; they need host cells to do it for them. All the same, they are very successful and we do not as yet have any medical magic bullet to fire at them – there is no viral antibiotic.

Our first line of defence against viruses is interferon. This is present in the blood in an inactive form all the time, but when faced with a virus it stimulates cells around it to make an active protein. This protein prevents the viral genetic material from being copied by host cells and so, in effect, stops the spread of the virus. It does, however, have a similar effect on our body cells, which is why it is not active all of the time; it is not specific and cannot choose which cells it stops, so viral particles, infected host cells and healthy cells are all fair game.

Whilst the viruses that cause mumps, measles, smallpox, herpes, polio, typhus and yellow fever are still in the blood, antibodies can attack them. The success of the viruses, however, depends on their ability to get inside host cells. Once inside a host cell they can be replicated, i.e. the host cell makes many more of them. The host cell also protects them from recognition by most of the immune army. Antibodies are no longer able to trap them. They in effect play one of the oldest tricks in the book – the Trojan horse. The only immune cell capable of recognising and killing viruses inside cells is the cytotoxic T cell.

Some viruses stay in the body even after obvious infection has passed, and can cause different symptoms when reactivated for some reason. The herpes group of viruses are a good example. The initial symptoms of infection clear up, but then after a low period, due perhaps to illness or stress, they reappear again; the chickenpox virus presents itself as shingles when it reappears. It has been suggested that reactivation of measles-type virus could be a cause of multiple sclerosis, but this is by no means definite.

The rhinoviruses (cold and flu viruses) are very successful, because they change their antigenic code quite often, i.e. the code that antibodies recognise does not remain the same. It is a bit like changing the buttons on a coat; the coat remains the same, but it appears different because of the buttons. The immune system remembers the 'button' code from the previous colds, but the cold you catch the next month has different buttons. So the B lymphocytes have to start all over again making new jackets to fit the 'new' virus. These viruses would be called clever if they had brains. In addition to this ability to put on disguises, they have other adaptations designed to get around the body's immune barriers, e.g. putting the respiratory tract cilia out of action. On top of that, the infection is relatively mild and both host and virus usually live to see another day (the host, however, being less than happy about the relationship).

The usually mild german measles virus can do severe damage to an under four-month-old foetus, and viruses like those causing AIDS and rabies are often fatal. Measles, mumps and glandular fever viruses cause immune suppression; in people who already have immune problems, these can be the last straw that breaks the camel's back. The mumps virus, for example, can cause autoimmune damage to the adult testis if the immune system is unable to halt the spread of the infection to that area. Cytomegalovirus infections and shingles can also be indicative of such immune suppression or deficiency.

DEALING WITH PROTOZOA

Less than 20 protozoa cause disease in man, but three of the insect-borne ones make very formidable enemies – the malarial parasite, injected by mosquitoes, Leishmania, spread by sandflies, and trypanosomes, causing sleeping sickness and carried by the tsetse fly. They have many tricks up their single-celled sleeves, but one has to be impressed by the trypanosomes as they have over 1,000 different buttons for their coats. They can change their distinguishing code so many times that it is unlikely to present the same sort of 'buttons' more than once. The immune system does not stand a chance of recognition.

DEALING WITH WORMS

Worms do not reproduce in man; they need another host as well, for example the pig in the case of tapeworms.

Antibody and eosinophils are the main immune soldiers to become involved in dealing with worms, although, because of the size of worms in comparison to bacteria and viruses, there are a lot of worm/antibody complexes.

Toxocariasis is one worm infection that causes concern in this country, as it is passed to humans via the cat or the dog. Pets should therefore be wormed regularly, especially if they are in contact with children. Toxocara larvae burrow into the blood vessels in the intestine; they then get to the liver, and are usually filtered out, but sometimes they get to the lungs, eyes or brain where, although they die, they can cause severe problems.

Threadworms cause anal irritation and are quite common in children of all races.

DEALING WITH FUNGI

Quite a number of different fungi can infect us. Dermatophytes, of which ringworm is one, are fungal infections found on the skin as a consequence of inadequate sebaceous secretions, too much soap, bubble baths, etc., or anything else which disturbs the acid and bug balance on the skin. A few fungi cause lung disease like aspergillus and cryptococcus.

Probably the most well known and increasingly common fungal infection is candida or thrush. Candida, in balance with bacteria and other organisms, is usually a harmless inhabitant of the gut and mucous membranes. But it has always been observed that undernourished, immunosuppressed and immunodeficient people suffer with symptoms directly attributed to candida, in particular if they have low levels of polymorphs or T cells.

Administration of antibiotics, whilst killing bacteria, favour overgrowth of candida, as do steroids. It is, of course, like any infection, catching; if genital thrush is the problem, there is little point treating one sexual partner without treating the other. Candida will always take advantage of any weak immune system and is always an accompanying infection in AIDS; not because it has anything to do with the cause of the disease, but because it is always first in line to take over when defence is weakened. Alcoholics and diabetics are also more prone to its attack because of weakened defences. Whether you blame excessive use of antibiotics or a general decline in the functioning of the immune system of people in this country is irrelevant to the statistical fact that candida infection is on the rapid increase, and is causing many problems.

Persistent fungal infections, and hence production of antibody complexes, can lead to a build up of granulomas which eventually calcify and may give joint problems – rheumatic-type pains.

VACCINATION

In general, then, we respond to an infection by using natural, active immunity. Vaccination, or artificial active immunity, is how medicine has used the body's own immune system to prevent disease. It was, and still is, a major medical tool and has led to the virtual eradication of smallpox from the world.

It is now a well-known story how Jenner inoculated a boy on the arm with material from a cowpox lesion. Two months later the boy was exposed to smallpox, but he did not develop the disease. Jenner had noticed that milkmaids who had cowpox never contracted smallpox; the cowpox bug – which was not fatal, unlike smallpox – made the body immune to smallpox. The World Health Organisation's smallpox programme has almost eradicated this disease, and it is no longer necessary to be vaccinated against it in this country. However, there may be a few isolated pockets in other areas of the world; Ethiopia was thought to be clear in 1976, while in 1963 Somalia was given a clean bill, although smallpox did raise its ugly head there again in the late 1970s.

Vaccines against bacteria causing tuberculosis, typhoid, whooping cough, cholera, diphtheria and tetanus, and against viruses causing smallpox, measles, polio, yellow fever, typhus and flu, are commonly available. There are others which may be provided for special circumstances, but which are not so readily available. It is interesting that one of the organisms which causes tooth decay is *Streptococcus mutans*, and it is hoped that a vaccine can be made against this organism, thus possibly preventing a lot of tooth decay.

Vaccines are made using:

- Modified bacterial toxins, e.g. diphtheria and tetanus.
- Killed organisms, e.g. whooping cough, polio.

- Living organisms, altered so that they cannot multiply and cause diseases, e.g. BCG vaccine for TB.

The successful use of vaccines has led to their routine use on the population in general. This is known as the immunisation programme.

Immunisation programmes

There is a lot of controversy about immunisation, and in the long run it comes down to a personal choice. The immunisation programme has been responsible for completely eradicating smallpox and it is marvellous to be able to use a technique which will stimulate the immune system to be resistant to such deadly bugs. However, I do have reservations about using it as a general routine or for illnesses which are not life threatening, as I think it is possible to over-stimulate the system. I also think that it is necessary to give the immune system normal practice at combating infection.

I am using the first person, I, throughout this section as this is only my personal view. Many, from both sides of the centre, will disagree and I do not know that anybody is right. Each individual needs to weigh up the pros and cons of each injection, depending on their own circumstances. I chose not to give my children the whooping cough vaccine, for example. They are both very healthy, active children, who are rarely sick. They throw off occasional infections very quickly, with hardly any signs at all that they are ill. I can be home to look after them if they are ill and I did not wish to take the risk of an adverse reaction. A mother who has to go out to work, whose child is in a large toddler group or playschool and who gets ill easily, may make the opposite choice. Similarly, measles and flu would be a minor irritation to my children and neither I nor they would have these injections. I do consider a tetanus jab is a good idea though, because the bug is freely available in the soil and children do play in the garden a lot.

Immunisation has its place. When it is needed it is very beneficial, but there are many possible side effects. The correct balance is again the key. We want an immune system which is supplied with the correct weapons to fight the battles in hand, not those it may never meet or that it can easily beat. The immune system should neither be under-supplied nor over-stimulated, just controlled and efficient.

Contraindications for immunisation are:
- If a person is unwell.
- If a woman is pregnant.
- If there has been any previous adverse reaction to a vaccine.

- If there is any history of fits.
- Live vaccines should not be given to those with malignant disease, especially if they are being given steroid or cytotoxic therapy.

IMMUNITY TO INFECTIOUS DISEASES

Overall, this will depend on a number of factors:
- Boosting active immunity artificially by means of immunisation.
- Boosting passive immunity artificially – providing short-term protection by giving antibodies or antitoxins if necessary.
- By keeping the disease-causing bugs out of the country, e.g. rabies, malaria, smallpox and yellow fever, and not allowing them to become endemic.
- By avoiding contact wherever possible, e.g. keeping sick children away from school or playschool and especially by keeping a six- to twelve-month-old baby away from playschools or older children with coughs, in the hope of avoiding whooping cough.
- Good hygiene standards are also important in preventing infections.
- By breastfeeding, in order to pass on maximum passive immunity to the baby in its first six months of life.
- By nutritionally boosting your active immune system at the first sign of infection, and preferably before any signs have appeared so as to help fend off invasion. This is achieved by consuming a low-fat, high-nutrient diet, avoiding processed foods and supplementing the key nutrients vitamin C (see page 142), beta-carotene, zinc, calcium and magnesium.
- By maintaining yourself as fit and healthy as possible most of the time, and keeping your immune enemies to the minimum.

8
AUTOIMMUNE DISEASES

We tend to think of man as having no predators. Under most circumstances man considers himself superior to lions, snakes and other 'lesser animals' that might try to kill him. Especially in this country, where the only place he is liable to meet any dangerous animals is at the zoo, man feels safe. Our main threat to individual survival – apart from ourselves, with our war games and supertoys like cars and planes – is from the microscopic living world. Fortunately for us, and through no design of our own, we have a complex immune system which puts up a very good fight against all foreign would-be intruders.

The fundamental characteristic of our immune system is that it does not normally take up arms against its own men and its own body. Autoimmunity is an outbreak of civil war in which this fundamental law is broken. There are several theories as to what happens, how the immune system recognises itself and how things go wrong to cause autoimmunity.

THE THEORIES

The immune language

Although our cells obviously cannot speak or write, they can use amino acid markers rather like we use letters of the alphabet. The immune system does not have sentences, only words, and so there are more words in the immune language than we are used to using. An average English-speaking person will have around 100,000 words available to them, although will only use a very small proportion of them. The immune system can synthesise around 10 million 'words'. In theory, antibodies can be made to each of these 10 million 'words'. However not everyone can synthesise all of these antibodies; some people have large gaps in their vocabulary. Autoimmunity is, in effect, a language problem, a misunderstanding caused by a lack of effective communication.

Just as it is impossible to communicate effectively with a lot of people at a party whilst they are all discussing different topics, so an overcrowded immune system also causes chaos. A well-ordered immune system is more like a small dinner party where it is possible to communicate effectively with everyone and everyone can join in the conversation and put forward their own views at some point.

The self marker theory

The thymus is the main computer for the immune army. It programmes some cells to be cytotoxic, others to have a role merely as regulators, and somehow it programmes immune cells to recognise self.

One possibility is that, from before the time of birth, the thymus lists markers on all of the cells belonging to self. Each different cell will have a different code or name, but our immune cells are programmed to recognise our own immune 'words' and to leave us alone. They only attack foreign words.

As with any complex system, there are loopholes. One is where a foreigner comes into the body, but has the same code as one of your cells, rather like an Australian or American whose native language is also English. The immune system recognises the language and leaves the foreigner alone. Some bugs like Treponema mimic an 'English word'; for a while such a bug is not attacked, as the immune cells recognise it as self. Then, when the body finally does realise that it is something with this 'word' that is causing all the problems, it attacks not only the bug but also the cells or tissues that have the 'word' on them that the bug has mimicked; in the case of Treponema, the immune system also turns against the heart-muscle cells containing cardiolipin. Therefore, the earlier that Treponema can be detected and killed with medical drugs, the less heart damage there will be. Streptococci A also have an antigen or marker or 'word' in common with another self marker, or 'word', on heart tissue; these strep bugs are associated with rheumatic fever. In many cases of this disease, anti-heart antibodies produced by our immune system cause heart damage.

It is also possible that ulcerative colitis is caused by confusion between an antigen or 'word' on a bug sometimes found in the gut, *E. coli*, and a marker or 'word' on the cells of the colon (large intestine). The presence of this bug causes the immune system to attack both the bug and the colon cells with the similar antigenic marker, resulting in inflammation and damage to the colon wall.

Another loophole is where a foreigner gets into a safe (English speaking) house before it is recognised, such as when a virus gets inside a host cell. The cytotoxic T cells get a bit blasé and carry on destroying those host cells, whether the cells have the foreigner inside or not. This is the body's own immune cells attacking itself, i.e. autoimmunity. So viral infections, in particular, can possibly cause autoimmunity years later.

Another example of a hidden antigen is sperm in a man's body. Sperm was not present in the young body when fluids and tissues were labelled as self. They developed later and thus are not actually recognised as self by the body – they are marked foreign. They are therefore 'hidden' from the immune system. In a rare complication of mumps, it is thought that the virus manages to attack the membranes separating the sperm from the rest of the body and the immune cells get in, fail to recognise the sperm as self and attack. Protein from the lens of the eye is similarly not recognised as self, and can be attacked by your own immune army if exposed to it.

The clonal theory

This theory suggests that we have the ability to make all antigens before birth, but that the thymus somehow turns off the ability to make antibodies to the codes which represent self; either it forgets to turn some antibodies off or they get switched on again to cause auto-immunity.

Which theory is correct?

It really makes little difference which theory is correct. The fact is that our immune cells have the ability to recognise self and not to attack it. They also have the ability to recognise an enemy and to attack it. Aging, pollution and bugs can alter our immune system so that it thinks that some cells marked self are enemies. Immune cells can also be changed so that they no longer recognise self codes and either leave everything alone, as in immune suppression, attack everything in sight, or attack the wrong thing.

The aim has to be to try to keep the immune army competent and accurate. So the enemies at any one time need to be kept to a minimum and the army must be provided with all the nutritional and other weapons it needs to be effective.

SOME AUTOIMMUNE CONDITIONS

There are quite a few autoimmune conditions, some of which are quite rare. The following is by no means a complete list, just examples of the more common ones. Interestingly, autoimmune diseases are much more common in women than in men.

Haemolytic anaemia

This is a form of anaemia (shortage of red blood cells) caused by an increase in red cell destruction, often in turn caused by self antibodies. It can sometimes be induced by drugs; if a drug attaches itself to red blood cells, the body's immune system attacks not only the drug but also its own cells. Penicillin can sometimes cause this, and so can some viruses. Fortunately, the instruction not to destroy itself is usually dominant and we do not all get haemolytic anaemia after flu or after the administration of penicillin.

Pernicious anaemia

Pernicious anaemia can be a result of autoimmune destruction of factors in the gut (parietal cells or intrinsic factor) which are involved in the uptake of vitamin B_{12}. If vitamin B_{12} is not absorbed, red blood cells are not formed in adequate numbers.

Addison's disease, diabetes and other endocrine disorders

Addison's disease (deficiency of the adrenal glands), diabetes and other endocrine disorders are often observed in patients with autoimmunity to the thyroid gland or gut. It should be mentioned, however, that most diabetes is not of the autoimmune type; adult onset diabetes is often due to a lifelong incorrect diet and does not involve auto-antibodies.

Systemic lupus erythematosus

Systemic lupus erythematosus, or SLE, is where auto-antibodies are made to genetic material (DNA and RNA). This makes the disease difficult to define in terms of symptoms as DNA and RNA are found in every living cell – almost any tissue may be attacked.

Rheumatoid arthritis

Rheumatoid arthritis is characterised by auto-antibody to IgG. As we have seen, IgG is a very common antibody and one which increases with age. The joint damage characteristic of the disease is probably caused by antigen/antibody complexes deposited in the joints; the damage is slowly progressive as the complexes build up.

There is another form of this disease which may be caused by an infection, viral or protozoan. Food sensitivity is often a contributory factor, rather than a causative agent, the most common trigger foods being meat or wheat.

9
IMMUNE-RELATED DISEASES

The immune system is usually successful in controlling microbial infections, simply because it can recognise a very large number of antigenic markers or 'words' and has some very strong weapons, in the shape of antibodies, chemicals and cells, which it can employ as and when necessary. These advantages can, however, also bring problems.

THE PROBLEMS

We have seen how antibodies can actually be turned to attack self, such that autoimmunity results. Furthermore, these antibodies and chemicals can also form complexes which cause disease.

A third disadvantage is the problem of transplant rejection, when we actually want a foreign non-self organ to be accepted as self in order to take the place of a faulty or worn-out piece of body.

Another problem is where the strong chemicals our immune system uses to kill bugs spill over or are released at the wrong time, and damage our own cells. This is often called hypersensitivity.

Lastly there are immune deficiencies, where for some reason the body cannot defend itself adequately.

Immune complex diseases

Infectious diseases and some autoimmune diseases like SLE (systemic lupus erythematosus) and rheumatoid arthritis form antigen/antibody complexes where the bug and antibody lock together. Usually macrophages or polymorphs come along and eat up the whole complex. Sometimes though – often through nutritional deficiency – the macrophage or polymorph gobbles up the complex but cannot digest it. Granulomas then form; these are fibrous and often calcified tissue containing material which the body cannot dispose of. It is an attempt at healing, rather in the same way as we put some toxic wastes into concrete cases before disposing of them.

Inflammation occurs around such complexes and is a characteristic of these diseases.

Granulomas cause problems if they cannot be stored satisfactorily. Diseases like sarcoidosis cause nodules in the lung, skin, eye, etc., and an increase in antibody but a deficiency in T cells.

Transplants

Organ transplants or skin grafts are likely to be attacked because the body does not recognise them as self. Success depends on matching the markers or 'words' on the transplant tissue as well as possible with the self markers, so that the immune system mounts the least hostile reaction, and then to suppress the immune system itself.

Some tissues cause more of an immune fuss than others. Kidney and bone marrow grafts can be quickly rejected by the immune system, the latter in particular always requiring a lot of immunosuppression if they are to be successful. Reaction to liver and hormone-forming organs is nowhere near as violent, and cornea and cartilage can usually be transplanted relatively easily.

Immunosuppression, if required, is brought about by drugs or by total body irradiation which knock out the cells of the immune system.

Hypersensitivity

Hypersensitivity is usually used to indicate allergy. This will be dealt with in Chapter II.

Immune deficiency

This may be the result of a genetic defect or malnutrition. If the defect is in the T cells, you become susceptible to viral and fungal infections, tumours and autoimmunity. In Hodgkin's disease and in Di George syndrome there is an almost complete absence of T cell activity, although antibody production, and hence control of bacteria, are normal. Patients with these diseases suffer with fungal and viral infections. In sarcoidosis and Crohn's disease there is a depression of T cell activity, but again the B cells are normal.

If the defect is in complement protein or B cells, bacterial infection and allergy are more likely, but autoimmunity could still be a problem. Deficiency of B cell activity for whatever reason gives rise to various forms of hypogammaglobulinaemia, i.e. a low level of antibody production; if macrophage and polymorph activity is compromised, granulomas result.

Progeria is a disease of the immune system characterised by vastly accelerated aging; a child with progeria looks like a little old man. It has been found that the eosinophil count in people with this disease is only 16 per cent of the total cell population, while it should normally be no lower than 31 per cent. The eosinophils are one type of white cell soldier and the eosinophil count always decreases with age. So keep the count up to stay youthful.

To be exact, everyone could be said to be immunodeficient at some time during their lives. Babies have immature immune systems. The elderly have less effective immune systems. Malnutrition, whether it be too much or too little of the major nutrients (calories, protein, fat, carbohydrates) or the micronutrients (vitamins, minerals, etc.) can cause a change in the immune response, as can an excess of anti-nutrients. Nutrients are capable of increasing numbers and activity of immune cells, while deficiencies can cause a slump in numbers and activity. But they can also prevent phagocytosis and the ability of phagocytes to digest their prey; they can interfere with fever control, and the production of interferon and other essential chemicals. Anti-nutrients block many necessary chemical steps and cause problems, wherever they are stored.

AIDS

Acquired immune deficiency syndrome (AIDS), caused by the human immunodeficiency virus (HIV), is probably the most well known immunodeficiency disease at present. The virus which causes the disease is rather like the flu virus in that it can change its coat repeatedly, so making it difficult for our natural immune system to recognise it again and difficult for us to make a vaccine against it. Unlike the flu virus, however, it makes a point of attacking the cells of the immune system itself – the T_4 cells. B cell activity is often normal or even above normal in AIDS patients; it is the T cells which suffer. The AIDS virus attacks the T helper cells which normally switch on the immune attack. This causes a relative excess of T suppressor cells which are the ones that turn the immune system off. The immune system is thus effectively turned off by the excess T suppressor cells, even though the body is under heavy attack.

The T cell deficiency means that the host is prone to many viral and fungal infections. Indeed, those who die with full blown AIDS are actually killed by the other opportunistic infections which move in, and not by the AIDS virus itself. However, some people with otherwise healthy immune systems, but who are infected with HIV, appear to be able to hold off the disease for a considerable time. If carrying the virus, anything which causes immunosuppression should obviously be avoided.

There is now a lot of information on AIDS and how to avoid it, so it will not be covered in detail here. The obvious prevention is to avoid the exchange of body fluids with an individual with the HIV virus, whether they have AIDS or not.

IMMUNITY TO TUMOURS

Tumour cells are cells that have turned traitor. It is almost as though they have decided to rebel, do their own thing, spread into whatever space they want, regardless of how this cramps other cells. People who already have a deficient or suppressed immune system will be much more susceptible to tumour formation.

Some tumours form spontaneously, one of the characteristics being a change in the way the cell 'breathes'. It no longer uses oxygen for obtaining energy; it switches to an anaerobic (non-oxygen using) metabolism. In today's highly chemicalised world, we have a lot of carcinogenic agents (chemicals which can induce tumours) in our environment and food.

At the time of writing, for example, Alar has just been banned. Alar was used on apples to make them all ripen at the same time and to keep them crisp for up to a year, but it has now been found to be one of the most potent carcinogens known. The additive 924, potassium bromate, has also been banned as a flour bleaching agent for use in bread. It was first found that it could cause nausea, stomachache, diarrhoea and even convulsions; further research showed that it destroyed vitamin E and caused cancer. These are only two examples out of a list of over 3,800 food additives. How many more will be found to have adverse effects on our immune systems?

These, and all our other manmade carcinogens, force us to cope with more enemies than is necessary. Macrophages can prevent the growth of some tumours, and interferon may do the same. NK or natural killer cells are small cells that we know relatively little about, but they also appear to be able to destroy some tumour cells, even without the help of antibodies, while the K or killer cells can do this as long as IgG antibody coats the tumour cells first. Complement, by way of the alternative pathway, is also thought to play a major part in tumour control. As this pathway is calcium independent, but magnesium dependent, it makes sense to ensure you get sufficient of this often deficient element.

There is no doubt whatever that any lumps or bumps which could, but may well not, be cancerous should be seen by a doctor and, if necessary, treated as soon as possible. There are very high success rates noted for the treatment of tumours, so the following chapter should not be taken as some sort of self-treatment for the condition; diet, however, may play a large part in the cause or prevention of cancer, as well as in its treatment, along with conventional therapy. It deserves a chapter to itself because of the high incidence of cancer in this country and because it allows us to take positive steps to avoid the condition.

10
DIET, IMMUNITY, TUMOURS AND CANCER

Cells in human tissue are characterised by regulated, limited growth. Sometimes, however, they will divide without restraint, the masses so formed being called tumours. Many tumours, like warts and other growths, are benign, not doing any harm. Other growths are or become malignant; their growth becomes invasive and causes damage.

There are many different types of cancer. That of the lymphoid tissue is called a lymphoma. If it is in the fleshy epithelial tissue it is a sarcoma; in the glands it is an adenocarcinoma; on the skin it is a melanoma; in the blood it is a leukaemia; and so on.

We do not know exactly what causes any type of cancer. Whilst smoking is strongly linked to cancer of the lung, a few people seem to be able to get away with smoking without developing the disease. Whilst sunlight and UV sunbeds are linked to skin cancer, the majority of people can benefit from exposure to the sun without developing the condition. The good news is that there are obviously other contributory factors to the development of a cancer apart from the primary factor; hopefully, diet, lifestyle and immune fitness can therefore play a part in the prevention of the disease.

VIRUS-INDUCED CANCER

The first evidence of viruses as the cause of some cancers was documented in 1908, when it was discovered that a certain type of chicken leukaemia could be transmitted by giving blood from diseased animals to healthy animals. Later it was found that the virus which was thought to cause mammary tumours in mice could similarly be passed on to their babies in their breast milk.

The main feature of viral-induced cancers is that, although they may have been transmitted at birth or in early childhood, they do not develop until adulthood, usually after childbearing age. Not only that, but they may not develop at all, even when there is medical evidence for the presence of the virus; some viruses manage to transform every cell they infect into a cancer, whilst others may infect many cells, but only one cell in 10,000 or so will be transformed. Some viruses known to cause cancer are the Epstein-Barr virus, the hepatitis B virus and the human T cell leukaemia virus.

Although some human cancers may well be of viral origin, no one has succeeded in isolating a virus from a human cancer and making it cause further cancers. Although there may be a familial link in some cancers, perhaps merely by perpetuating the same diet or lifestyle, human cancer is not considered to be 'catching'. The condition of the immune system is obviously vitally important in the prevention of viral-induced cancers.

HOW ELSE DOES CANCER START?

Although the eventual development of cancer appears to be influenced by many contributory factors, there is often one specific stimulus which triggers the whole process. This trigger may be anything which upsets the body's chemical balance and causes irritation of the cells and an increased growth rate. Alcohol, aflatoxins (mould poisons), smoking, pesticides, food additives, environmental pollutants, radiation, domestic and industrial chemicals are examples of potential triggers which alone, or in combination, could upset our biochemistry. Nutrient deficiencies or excesses, hormonal upsets, inappropriate exercise and unfulfilled emotional needs could also be contributory factors. The key to avoiding cancer is to get the balance right.

ACID/ALKALINE BALANCE

If a weak acid is added to cells, their growth is slowed down. If a weak alkaline solution is added however, cells are stimulated to grow faster. When we are in normal good health our blood and lymph are slightly alkaline (pH 7–7.4) and our urine is slightly acid (except after a meal containing a lot of protein when it may be temporarily slightly alkaline). It is important to maintain the body's normal acid/alkaline balance. If the body becomes too alkaline, cancerous growth is favoured.

SALT

Salt, in excessive amounts, gets the blame for many disease conditions, including our number one killer, heart disease. There is also a very good theory as to why it should also be a causative agent in our number two killer, cancer.

It is widely acknowledged that the Western diet contains too much salt (sodium chloride). Even people who do not add salt directly to their food fall prey to the vandal, sodium, which is hidden in our processed foods.

Commercially prepared bread can contain a lot of salt, wholemeal often contains more than white bread. Salted butter too can have around half a teaspoon of salt to every ounce. Most processed foods have a high salt content, either as a raising agent or preservative, or for flavouring. All cooked and processed meats like sausages and bacon, tinned fish in brine, smoked foods and many cheeses are high in salt. Other sodium compounds like sodium bicarbonate are consumed in such foods as soda bread and sponges, or may even be taken as an antacid or to give drinks a fizz. A high intake of such foods puts us on the sodium merry-go-round; it makes us deficient in zinc which in turn reduces our sense of taste. This causes us to crave for even saltier and tastier foods. The sodium, being very reactive, displaces other elements from the body, in particular calcium, and this causes muscular weakness, flabbiness, low energy levels, constipation and a weakened pulse rate. All of these symptoms are likely to be found in a cancer patient.

A cancer cell differs from an ordinary body cell in that it grows abnormally fast, has an excess of alkalinity, a low calcium content and an anaerobic (without oxygen) form of respiration.

Sodium is believed to be a factor in cancer because an excess of it will encourage cells to exhibit all of these factors. Excess sodium will form caustic soda – a strong irritant alkali – in the body. The increased alkalinity causes cells to reproduce faster, in order to produce more lactic acid in an attempt to rectify the situation. Calcium is turned out of the cells by the sodium. Free sodium is very reactive and must combine with something and will often rob the red blood cells of their carbon dioxide in order to make carbonate of soda. Unfortunately red blood cells need their carbon dioxide to swap it for oxygen in the lungs. If their carbon dioxide is reduced, so is their ability to pick up vital oxygen needed by our tissues.

The salt connection is still a theory but if it is right many cancers could be prevented by adjusting the diet to give the correct acid/alkaline balance and reducing the sodium in the diet to the amount necessary for good health.

As an excess of sodium is also implicated in causing heart disease, reducing sodium intake seems to be a very sensible and safe precaution to take. Taste buds do eventually adjust, and foods which are too salty become unpleasant. At best, you have taken a safe and simple step towards the prevention of cancer and heart disease; at worst you have merely saved yourself the cost of the salt.

Interestingly, sunshine does not seem to induce skin cancer unless there is an excess of sodium in that person. Soap should not be left on the skin as it is basically sodium salt of an organic acid (just as common salt is that of an inorganic acid).

SMOKING

If you smoke, the risk of heart disease, cancer and various other ailments is increased. The only real solution is to give it up, or perhaps not start in the first place. Whilst you are doing this, or if you really cannot or do not wish to give up, extra supplements of beta-carotene and vitamin C are advisable.

DIET

Many authorities agree that a faulty diet is one of our leading contributory factors in the causation of cancer and heart disease. Our main problem is that of over-eating, in particular too many calories or too much fat. Being too fat is a greater risk factor in women, as it causes the body to produce more oestrogen. The good news is that it is never too late to start restricting your diet; animal studies have shown that restricted feeding, even after cancer formation, slows its growth.

Nutrient deficiencies are also considered to be contributory factors, in particular deficiencies of vitamins C, E, and beta-carotene.

VITAMIN C

It is interesting that most animals can make their own vitamin C, and do so in greater quantities when they are ill. Man has lost this ability to synthesise vitamin C and needs to obtain it from his diet.

In 1954, a German doctor reported that ten terminally ill cancer patients had been given larger doses of vitamins A and C – in the order of grams – and their tumours shrank and shrank. This study was extended to 100 patients and the results were confirmed. Many other researchers have since obtained similar results but the difficulty in getting consistent confirmative results with such supplements is that everyone is different – the dose is crucial but varies from person to person. The vitamin C dose for example, is usually taken as just under the amount needed to cause diarrhoea; the individual gradually increases the vitamin C intake to the point where they experience diarrhoea, and then they go back a gram or two and maintain that dosage.

Perhaps cancers are caused by dietary deficiencies (or excesses) on top of a primary attacker like a virus, smoke, a chemical additive or excess radiation. This would explain why vitamin C therapy works for some people but not for others, why beta-carotene works for some but not for others, etc. To help prevent cancer it is therefore wise to ensure plenty of beta-carotene- and vitamin C-containing foods; but remember that a fresh orange may have about 180 mg of vitamin C, whereas a stored one may not have any at all. If you are in doubt about the sources of natural vitamin C in foods and fruit, it might be necessary to consider a reliable food supplement. When such supplemental vitamin C is required, pure ascorbic acid powder is best as it contains no fillers or binders necessary to make up tablets, and can be stirred into orange juice or water. However some people cannot take the acidity of ascorbic acid and these people may require calcium ascorbate; sodium ascorbate is not the best choice for a supplement due to its sodium content.

Vitamin C and the skin
Vitamin C can also be used to protect the skin. A few grains in the bath water or sink is probably better than soap, at least for a final rinse, as it leaves the skin slightly acid. (Better still, take a bath with a lemon. It smells good too.) There are a few reports that claim the clearing of skin tumours with local and oral vitamin C – worth trying on non-malignant tumours like warts if they keep reappearing after being burned or surgically removed.

Any tumours which have become cancerous should, of course, be given immediate medical attention. The success rate for halting melanomas (malignant skin tumours) is very high if they are caught early enough, but they invade quickly and it must be stressed that anyone should not *think* too long about it before going to the doctor with a growing, bleeding or weeping mole. Go right away.

What else does vitamin C do?

- Cancerous degeneration of cells is preceded by a softening of tissue and a loss of collagen, the connective tissue. One of vitamin C's chief functions is the formation of this hard collagen. So perhaps if we had enough vitamin C, the softening would not occur.
- Hard cancer of the breast is less invasive than soft breast cancers, and again vitamin C can be crucial in making harder tissue.
- Vitamin C kills viruses in the laboratory and is required by the body's immune army for producing weapons against viruses. So a steady intake of vitamin C is protective against all viruses, including the possible cancer-causing ones.
- Lymphocytes need vitamin C to move towards an invader, to engulf it and to produce the chemicals to digest it. Interferon also requires vitamin C.
- Vitamin C (ascorbic acid) is acidic and can therefore help to neutralise excess alkalinity often caused by excessive salt intake.
- Nitrite, which is unfortunately common in our diet and is also a common constituent of several drugs, can be turned into nitrosamines in the body. These are carcinogenic. Vitamin C prevents this change from occurring.
- In the laboratory vitamin C blocks transformation of cells into cancer cells, even in the presence of a cancer-causing substance, and it inhibits the division of cancer cells without affecting normal cells.
- One study of 169 women calculated that women whose daily intake of vitamin C was below the recommended daily allowance were ten times more likely to suffer from cervical abnormalities compared to those whose intake was over the allowance.
- Vitamin C taken before going to bed can be used as a preventative measure against bladder cancer, as the excess vitamin C remains in the bladder all night.

VITAMIN E

A high-fat diet and lack of vitamin E are associated with breast cancer in women. Fluid from breasts at risk have been found to contain high levels of lipid peroxides – really rancid fat. Smoking and other chemicals cause rancidity of fats, and the breast is a fatty tissue with relatively poor circulation, where such fats will collect and stagnate. Massage could be beneficial in preventing this stagnation and improving circulation.

Free radicals are chemical units formed under certain circumstances, in particular when polyunsaturated fats turn rancid. Their importance in this context is that their presence is thought to be a risk factor in many diseases, including cancer. The production of these free radicals is prevented by substances known as antioxidants – vitamins C and E are powerful antioxidants.

Vitamin E is a naturally occurring antioxidant found in many oils and fats, but during processing the vitamin E is often removed and is replaced by an artificial antioxidant. This is fine for preventing the fat going off while it's in the bottle, but not a lot of use once it gets into the body. Cold pressed oils are the best buy, but no oil should be kept too long or heated and reheated.

It would appear that women are more susceptible to cancer (especially breast cancer) from eating too many polyunsaturated fats whilst being deficient in vitamin E.

BETA-CAROTENE

Beta-carotene, the non-toxic precursor of vitamin A, is very effective in maintaining cell wall integrity, so keeping viruses out. It is being used in the treatment of some cancers and, although evidence is still controversial, it is worth maintaining good levels of this substance in the diet for the prevention of cancer. It is also worth taking it as a supplement if you have cancer, and particularly if you are an addicted smoker – beta-carotene may well be helpful in the prevention and treatment of lung cancer.

FIGHTING CANCER

Fighting cancer should become a team effort, with everyone playing their part to get the best result for the patient. Prevention of cancer, however, is up to you. You are responsible for going for screening or reporting lumps and bumps. Your lifestyle and diet can put you at risk or offer protection.

Cancer itself is like a team sport. If cancer only has one member of its team playing, it is unlikely to win, even if it is a very strong and skilful player (like salt or cigarette smoke); but as soon as other members of the cancer team join in (like dietary excesses, toxic minerals, lack of exercise, stress, etc.) the chances of cancer scoring a goal become much more likely.

If your immune team is good and strong, the score may well be a win to you or a draw at the end of play, but if your immune team start dropping out with injuries, the cancer team could win.

We must therefore aim to keep the cancer team low in number and maintain a full and well trained side on our immune system. Then we can surely win.

II
ALLERGY

Allergy occurs when the body alters its normal immune response in some way, due to the presence of an allergen. Allergens are substances which bring about this immune response, and the odd thing about them is that they are not normally harmful; it appears to be the allergic individual who produces the wrong response. Ironically, many allergy sufferers are immune deficient in other ways as well.

In the case of contact sensitivities, such as allergy to nickel, jewellery or detergents, it is the lymphocytes and macrophages which over-react, but in most other allergies it is the antibody response which is over-reactive. The role of antibodies in allergy was not really well known until 1967, when the antibody IgE was discovered and associated with hayfever. IgE is not produced all over the body; it is made mainly in nasal and throat areas and the gut. It is believed that cross-links between IgE molecules and the surface of our mast cells (mast cells are specialised immune cells dotted around our tissues, packed with immunologically active chemicals) and basophils cause the release of histamine, and it is the histamines, normally safely packaged inside the cells, which cause the soreness and itching and hence the need for anti-histamine medication. Vitamin C is a natural anti-histamine and can often be used to alleviate symptoms if the dose is right. IgA and IgG are also involved in allergic reactions.

Response to an allergen may be immediate or delayed, and is by definition an inappropriate or over-reaction of the immune system to inhaled or non-inhaled allergens. However, although a true allergy has to evoke an immune response, the term allergy is often broadened to include food intolerances.

WHO SUFFERS FROM ALLERGIES?

Whether due to an overall decline in our immune competence or to an increase in the burden on our immune system, or perhaps a bit of both, the cases of allergies are rapidly increasing.

Allergies can sometimes run in families. It is known that high total

IgE levels can be inherited, as can faulty T cell response. The allergy, however, may not be the same down the generations. A child with asthmatic parents may be more prone to allergy, but she may suffer with eczema or hayfever instead.

Allergic symptoms also change with age. A baby with eczema may grow out of it only to become an adult who suffers from hayfever. Children often appear to suffer more from allergy than adults, but this may not actually be true; it could merely be that we are more aware of a child's symptoms and they have less control over them. An adult has learned how to cope with his recurrent migraine, but a child will perhaps be sick, and frightened of how she is feeling.

COMMON ALLERGENS

Inhalant	Dust; animal furs; moulds; perfumes; pollen; industrial, domestic and agricultural chemicals; gas; smoke; exhaust fumes; air conditioner or propellant gases.
Contact	Nickel; jewellery; soaps and detergents; bleaches; other household or industrial chemicals; cosmetics; animals; paints and dyes; glues.
Non-inhalant	Bites and stings from insects, etc.; drugs, e.g. penicillin, aspirin; foods, especially fish, nuts, wheat, milk products, meat and eggs; artificial foods, especially colourings and flavourings.

COMMON ALLERGIC REACTIONS

These are usually grouped on the basis of the areas they affect.

The skin

Contact with an allergen can bring about various forms of dermatitis.

Hives

Hives are large whitish raised areas on the skin, with an itching red centre. They are often caused by a reaction to an insect bite, but they may be due to some other allergen. They sometimes come and go, in which case it is difficult to find the cause. The itching may be worse with exercise or any form of overheating including hot baths, tight clothes and emotional upset.

Eczema
This can be very itchy, and is usually worse in winter. It often starts as rough red patches on babies' cheeks; it may then disappear completely or come and go, spreading to other areas.

Wool can sometimes cause this or other types of skin reaction, but if the eczema persists there is nothing for it but to go through the whole list of possible allergens. It is helpful if you think back to the day before each incident occurred, particularly the first one.

It is far better to trace the cause of the eczema and remove it if possible, rather than resort to cortisone creams or other anti-histamines (which are all immunosuppressants), but this is not always practical. Bubble baths and soaps are also best avoided, except for washing the hands and nails. Laundry soap has to be a suspect, and it may be necessary to use pure soap suds only for washing and then to put the washing through the machine again with no soap at all – just water. Exposure to some viruses, especially the cold sore virus, herpes, can make eczema worse. Even a smallpox or similar vaccination could be a real problem. Food is often a cause of eczema, and food allergies are worth investigating (see the next chapter).

Eczema is especially bad for children, as they automatically scratch the itch, which makes it even worse and can cause infection. Keep the fingernails short and clean, and perhaps buy cotton gloves to prevent involuntary scratching at night.

The head
Allergic symptoms may affect the eyes, nose, ears, lips or brain.

Migraine
This region is very susceptible to allergic reactions. Some forms of migraine can be caused by allergy, but it is not easy to find the cause; there are different triggers for different people and no one solution that works for everyone. It seems that allergens may cause the blood platelets to slow down the blood flow to the head by clumping together. A migraine attack follows, often causing a one-sided headache with feelings of nausea. Some people suffer so badly that they are forced to lie in a darkened room and hope for sleep. Attacks may last for hours or even days.

There are whole lists of foods and chemicals which have been cited as potential triggers for migraine, the most common being cheese, chocolate, yeasts, food flavours and colours, red wine, coffee, tea and sugar. Some medicines, like the pill, and some household chemicals have also been implicated.

Headaches may also be brought about by constriction of the blood vessels in the neck region due to some misalignment of the vertebrae; if so, an osteopath may be required to correct the problems. Involuntary constriction of the blood vessels is another cause and can be prevented by ensuring sufficient magnesium and niacin in the diet. Platelets may aggregate, leading to headaches, but they can be kept separated by having enough vitamins E, C, B_6 and the essential fatty acids. Ensuring nutrient sufficiency and avoiding chemical triggers could avert many migraines. It all depends on the cause of the problem in the first place and, unfortunately, it often takes a lot of time and detective work to uncover the cause.

Hayfever

Hayfever causes a running nose, sneezing and watery eyes. Sufferers often have to clear their throat and breathe through the mouth; they may lose their sense of taste and smell to some degree. Hayfever can also cause altered moods, making people irritable, touchy, fussy, moody and listless; emotions can be involved, and children, in particular, cry very easily.

If you are a sufferer, things other than pollen to which you are sensitive may bring on an attack, even pets. There is one school of thought that links susceptibility to hayfever with high wheat and sugar consumption; both of these are in the same family as the pollen which is known to trigger hayfever in this country. Many sufferers, although by no means all, relieve symptoms by switching to an unrefined diet low in wheat and sugar products.

Hayfever can also cause swelling inside the nose, the membranes becoming stretched and less resistant to infection; infection of ears, nose and throat is thus often an additional problem. The swelling and pressure in the nasal tissue can impair blood circulation, so dark circles as well as puffiness under the eyes are common features. The weakened nasal tissue is also likely to break and bleed, causing nose bleeds. Polyps may develop, especially if the hayfever sufferer is also sensitive to aspirin and foods containing salicylates – many herbs, spices and alcoholic drinks are high in salicylates, as are tea, coffee, cola and yeast foods.

Asthma

Aspirin and beta-blocker (blood-pressure-lowering drugs) sensitivity is more common in asthmatics than other people. Asthmatics are also more sensitive to metabisulphite (the preservative in wine and squashes) and tartrazine, as well as to polyunsaturated fats. Hayfever can go on to develop into bronchial asthma, slipping, so to speak, from the nose to the chest. Asthma is not always due to allergy, but if the patient has previously suffered with eczema or hayfever, it probably is an allergic reaction. Most allergies are more common in females, but asthma is the exception, being two or three times more common in males.

Swelling occurs in the lining of the air tubes in the lung and the muscle around the air tube contracts, possibly due to an imbalance of calcium and magnesium in the diet; an asthmatic thus needs more dietary magnesium. With the swelling inside and squeezing outside, the air space in the tubes is much smaller and there is difficulty pushing the air out – hence the typical wheezing of asthma.

Wheezing causes a build-up of mucus in the lung. It is vital for an asthmatic to drink a lot, as this helps to keep the fluid thin; if it is allowed to become thick and rubbery, the problems get worse and may bring about vomiting, which in turn causes dehydration, so even more fluid is needed. It is important, however, not to drink things that will make this condition worse – ice-cold fluids, colas and coloured drinks can often cause problems.

Allergic symptoms may also affect other areas of the body, such as the hands, stomach, feet, blood vessels and bladder.

As with most allergic problems, it is a question of trying to find the triggers that bring about the condition. To complicate matters, there are often several triggers, not just one, which makes them not only difficult to find but also difficult to eliminate from the diet or immediate environment.

OTHER CONDITIONS THOUGHT TO BE ASSOCIATED WITH ALLERGY

Behaviour problems
Hyperactivity, vandalism and crime is going up all over the world and not just in proportion to the increase in population. Quite a few studies now show a link between diet and such antisocial behaviour (and it appears that unreal fears and phobias may also be associated with food or chemical sensitivity). Work has been done with prisoners and juvenile offenders which has shown that dietary modifications reduce aggressive and destructive behaviour. The link between allergies, nutritional imbalances and crime is only slowly being accepted in this country, but why are we so reluctant to accept what could be a very simple way to keep the crime rate down? We

readily accept that alcohol and drugs destroy the body's reason and control, so why not chemicals in or sprayed on to foods? Animals put on a diet where the natural food has been replaced by highly processed foodstuffs have consistently shown increased aggressive behaviour.

The classic example is that of an American who was allergic to a specific red wine. He went out to dinner one evening, drank some of this wine, then stood up and shot several people. He was, of course, arrested, but denied intending to shoot those people. He was hospitalised and tested by being given various drinks disguised as red wine. One day, they gave him the real stuff and he lost control and had to be restrained with a straightjacket. His reaction was real.

Our foods and environment, along with our immune responses to them, could have more to do with our behavioural as well as our medical problems than we realise. A lot more research needs to be done, but results to date look promising. The trouble is, it is a lot easier to tell a person to take a pill or two every day than it is to tell them to eliminate their favourite foods from their diet and to expect them to stick to it.

Alcoholism
Our tolerance of alcohol varies from individual to individual, but even the complete teetotaller has to cope with alcohol, and gets through roughly two measures of alcohol per day, though it never passes their lips (a measure of alcohol is equivalent to a glass of wine or half a pint of beer). Alcohol is made in all of us by the bugs that live in our gut and ferment our food; and people on a high sugar and refined food diet, and those with yeast infections in the gut, make more alcohol than the rest of the population.

The liver deals with the alcohol, releasing a zinc-dependent enzyme which renders it harmless. In a zinc-sufficient person with normal liver function one measure of alcohol is dealt with in roughly half an hour. When alcohol intake exceeds the body's ability to process it we get light-headed and then drunk.

Studies done with alcoholics now show that they often have sensitivities to wheat, corn, rye, malt, sugar or yeast. People without sensitivities to these related foods are less likely to become addicted to alcohol, even though they may drink a lot more than those who are.

Fits and heart problems
Ingestion of or exposure to food or chemical allergens can bring on fits, irregular heartbeats, high blood pressure, chest pains and blood

clots. Research is still relatively new and incomplete in this area, but there is the possibility that some strokes and heart-related problems could be avoided if only we could recognise our food and chemical sensitivities, deficiencies and excesses.

Inflammatory bowel diseases

Inflammatory bowel diseases like Crohn's disease and ulcerative colitis are often blamed on food sensitivities, but exclusive diets should not be undertaken without professional guidance, as people with gut problems are often already very nutrient deficient due to the inability of the gut to digest and absorb normally. Antibodies to cows' milk and salicylates are often found in someone with ulcerative colitis, but avoiding foods containing these does not always bring relief. Supplements (of zinc in particular) are often required.

Coeliac disease is a sensitivity to gluten (found in wheat and some other cereals), but may well include a sensitivity to the rest of the grains as well.

Arthritis

Arthritis comes in various different forms. It is really a term which covers several conditions that have similar effects on the joints, but there is no definite single cause. Treatment, likewise, varies and what may be a miracle cure for one person can have no effect at all on another.

Food and chemical allergies have been cited as major offenders in many cases of rheumatoid arthritis, with remarkable claims from people confined to wheelchairs who were able to get up and walk after eliminating certain foods like red meat or perhaps dairy products, wheat, tea or coffee from the diet. These foods have also been labelled as aggravators in cases of osteoarthritis. It should be mentioned that it is usually one or two of these major risk foods that are a problem and they vary from person to person. Exclusion diets will be considered in the next chapter, but they can be dangerous on a self-help basis if too much is left out.

Anti-inflammatory drugs are often prescribed to reduce the pain and swelling in arthritis, but they do nothing to make the disease any better. Dietary therapy can sometimes have an effect equal to, if not better than, these drugs. Zinc and copper are very important in reducing inflammation, but they need to be in balance, as they work together with manganese. If the balance of these three is right, inflammation is minimised. If they are out of balance, the pain increases. A copper bracelet seems to work very well for some arthritics, but others get an aggravation of symptoms or no effect at all as a result of wearing one. Probably the acidity of the skin dissolves small amounts of copper, which are then absorbed. If the patient has a low copper status, then additional copper brings relief. If, however, the copper is already high in this person and the zinc is low, there could be aggravation. This type of person may get relief from zinc supplementation, although the dose will be dependent on the individual. The fatty acids are the building blocks of fats, just as amino acids are the building blocks of proteins. We can synthesise most of the fatty acids we need, but there are three – arachidonic, linoleic and alpha-linolenic acids – that we are unable to manufacture and that are needed for a wide range of functions. We therefore have to ensure that these are provided in the diet. But that is not all; we also have to ensure that we receive these EFAs (essential fatty acids) in the right proportions. In particular, if the balance is tipped in favour of arachidonic acid, it appears to promote the production of substances called leukotrienes in the mast cells – and leukotrienes are many times more inflammatory than histamine. A reduction in the intake of saturated fats and an increased intake of the unprocessed polyunsaturates, particularly cold-pressed safflower oil, cod liver oil and EPA (eicosapentaenoic acid, a derivative of alpha-linolenic acid, and available as a supplement), swings the balance away from arachidonic acid and may well be of benefit in arthritis.

Poor mineral absorption is also often a contributory factor in arthritis. Diets that include tea and coffee, or bran with everything, should be avoided as these deplete vitamin and mineral absorption. A balanced supplement may be necessary, but make sure you consult someone who knows what they are doing, as you will be using nutritional supplements like drugs. For example, iron supplements should not be taken by anyone with any inflammatory condition such as arthritis.

12
FOOD SENSITIVITIES AND SLIMMING

A girl came to see me for nutritional advice. She looked dreadful, a sunken wreck. She was eating peanuts – that was all, nothing but peanuts. She believed that she was allergic to various different foods, and had been eliminating them one by one. By the time she came to see me she had given up everything except peanuts. A doctor from the eating disorder clinic at the Bristol Royal Infirmary confirmed that she was seeing other people doing the same sort of thing. It cannot be stressed enough that if you are slimming, or if you are trying to detect foods to which you are allergic, the more you restrict the variety of foods which you eat, the less balanced and more hazardous your diet is likely to be.

If you are slimming, 1,000 calories, 4,200 joules or 4.2 kilojoules per day should be the absolute minimum, and these calories must be carefully selected to give the range of nutrients needed. Medical supervision is needed for anything below this, and will probably be advised even at this level in many cases where there are additional conditions or problems.

To detect food allergies only one or two food groups should be tested at a time. If there are multiple allergies, professional supervision is needed to make sure that essential nutrients are replaced in some other form.

FOOD AND CHEMICAL SENSITIVITIES

Symptoms of food and chemical sensitivities are similar; indeed, the two often go hand in hand. For example, you may have no problem eating an organic apple or lettuce, but go into a spin after eating those that have been sprayed. If you find that you do have a reaction to a fruit, vegetable or grain, it is worth experimenting with the organic form just to make sure that it is not a reaction to a chemical used on the food.

Recent research has certainly shown that we can be allergic to, or become allergic to, everyday foods. Very often it is the foods that we have become addicted to and eat every day that cause the problems; hence the most common foods, such as wheat, eggs, sugar, milk and dairy produce, meat, tea and coffee, tend to be the ones that most often cause problems. We are not all sensitive to the same foods; each of us is different.

Symptoms of sensitivities

Initial symptoms of food sensitivities may be vague, even mild, but they can change enigmatically or get more persistent as life continues. Like alcohol and drugs, a food or chemical can become addictive and can eventually cause more serious and destructive symptoms. It first gives an uplifting sensation and creates a desire for it, but it also has its hangover – the depressed or low reaction, some of which are listed below.

- Skin reactions can include eczema, itching patches, dryness, hives.
- Head reactions can include headaches, migraines; dizziness; fear of heights; unreal sensations like floating or being detached; ringing or fluid in the ears, earache; sensitivity to light, dull itchy eyes, watery eyes; emotional instability, crying or edgy laughter; frequent throat clearing or cough, rhinitis, voice irregularities.
- Chest symptoms can include bronchitis, breathing difficulties; irregular or pronounced heart beat; high blood pressure.
- Gut and trunk problems can include stomachache or swelling; constipation or diarrhoea; indigestion, nausea, vomiting; water retention, frequency of urination, bedwetting, especially in children allergic to coloured lollies or drinks.
- Muscle and joint pains can include vague and perhaps mobile aches and pains; swelling of joints; muscle spasms; unusual weakness, progressing later into rheumatism or arthritis.
- General symptoms can include poor concentration, inability to think clearly; lack of energy; irritability or moodiness, perhaps progressing to depression and despair.

PREVENTING SENSITIVITY

The most desirable choice is to prevent sensitivity occurring, but it requires willpower. These suggestions are useful for preventing further problems.

- Eat raw foods before cooked food. When we eat, white blood cells line up along the gut wall, and it seems that raw food does not cause destruction of these white blood cells as much as cooked food. The French idea of *crudités* before a meal is a good habit to get into, and is also quite slimming.
- Avoid becoming addicted to any food by ensuring you don't eat the same item or items of food every day. If you are in good health and are not knowingly suffering from any allergy symptoms, one week in every ten without one's 'fix' may well be enough to prevent addiction. Milk is a common food to which we may become addicted if we suffer with a leaky gut because it is drunk in tea or coffee, providing little injections of it throughout the day, every day. Wheat, too, is a national addiction. Although we may think we have a varied diet, it is often only the added flavours and colours and the change of texture that is different. Bread, buns, cakes, pastries, pies, pasties, quiches, pizzas, batter, biscuits and breakfast cereals all contain wheat. It is, in fact, quite difficult to eliminate wheat entirely from the diet, because wheat is hidden in some form in many foods. There are many cereal grains that we could eat instead of wheat, and using them as part of the regular diet would improve our nutrition in more ways than one.
- Have a very varied diet, using, as far as possible, fruits, vegetables and fish in their seasons. It is now possible to buy some foods, strawberries for example, nearly all year round; but, while strawberries are delicious, it is very easy to get an allergic reaction from them. So enjoy them whilst they are in season and then leave them alone for a while. Never narrow foods down to a monotonous daily routine.
- Use wholefoods rather than highly processed and chemically treated foods where possible.

SENSITIVITY REACTIONS OF SOME FOODS

Stimulants

Some sufferers can easily become addicted to stimulants like tea, coffee, alcohol, nicotine, sugar, or simply overbreathing. When an allergen enters the stomach it causes a war, and histamine is released. This, in turn, causes more biochemicals to be released from the stomach and the whole body, including the brain, gets a flood of these. The brain reacts to the chemical stimulation and the result is a 'high' feeling which is easy and pleasant to become addicted to.

Nuts

To the immune system all nuts are similar and, having developed an allergy to one, it is easy to do the same for another. Nuts are the biggest seeds and in very sensitive people cause the tongue and throat to swell. Chocolate is a form of nut and so should be included in this category. Arthritics are often particularly sensitive to nuts and chocolate. It is unfortunate, as nuts are nutrient-packed foods, but it is necessary to rotate them in the diet.

Milk

It is possible to have an allergic reaction to cold milk but not to hot milk; this is due to an allergen which is destroyed on heating. This means that you may be able to drink milk which has been boiled.

A beef allergy does not have to go with a milk allergy, and cheeses have many different allergens in them unrelated to milk. So a cheese allergy does not necessarily rule out milk. And a milk allergic may well be able to eat butter, as milk fat and protein are different antigenically.

Fish

People allergic to bony fish (herring, mackerel, cod, haddock) may not be allergic to cartilaginous fish such as skate, ray, shark and dogfish, as the antigen is different. Similarly, the jointed and mollusc shellfish have different antigens.

Shellfish are especially well known for causing allergies as they have copper-containing enzyme systems and a substance called haemocyanin which is a very powerful antigen and makes a lot of people develop urticaria or be sick.

Fruit and vegetables
Allergic reactions from these are often due to chemicals sprayed on to them, but they do carry antigens of their own. Raw carrots and raw celery have a common antigen to which a few people become sensitive, but this is destroyed on cooking, so these individuals can eat cooked but not raw carrots and celery. Orange peel and apple pips have antigens which occasionally cause problems. Onions, leeks and garlic have quite strong-reacting antigens – often the stronger the taste, the stronger the antigen.

Yeast
Even the smell of bakers' yeast can set some people off, and they certainly cannot eat home-baked bread. However, they may well be able to tolerate shop bread, where the allergen has been denatured by greater heat.

Meat
Lamb is usually the least likely to cause an allergy problem. Pork is often a problem in asthmatics and beef in rheumatoid arthritics. Adults with eczema sometimes cannot eat meat at all without a reaction.

WHAT HAPPENS IN FOOD ALLERGY

Most people think that food is digested in the gut and is then absorbed into the bloodstream, but sometimes, it seems, incompletely digested food goes straight into the bloodstream. This is known as persorption, and happens more often in people with weak or damaged guts.

The immune soldiers in the bloodstream get rid of the undigested food, but in doing so they make antibodies to it, treating it as an antigen. This is often how food allergy starts. Once the antibodies are made to a food, the body is sensitised and makes more of them when that food is encountered next. The result is that antigen/antibody complexes are formed, some of which may go to the liver; but others are deposited in joint spaces where they activate neutrophils and release a powerful free radical called superoxide – hence the arthritis link with food sensitivities.

The worst way to deal with a food sensitivity is to have the offending food – the antigen or allergen – little and often, because there will then always be more antibody available than there is antigen. This causes antibody/antigen complexes to be formed, and the symptoms of food sensitivity result. A better way to deal with the problem is to have a lot of the offending food in one go, and then forget about it completely for a few days. The body only makes a small amount of antibody at any one time and if the food (the allergen) is in excess of the antibody, there are fewer antibody/ antigen complexes formed and less reaction. This is called masking.

Technically the gut is a tunnel running right through the body, and nutrients have to pass from the inside of the tunnel into the body. The immune system mounts little reaction to substances in the gut, i.e. in the tunnel, but a response will invariably be invoked if anything foreign – non-self – gets into the body through a faulty tunnel wall, without being processed first. The major lymphoid tissue in the gut is the Peyer's patches in the intestines, but there appears to be no such tissue above the level of the waist. In this region the principal immunological agent is IgA; this has limited biological activity, and no memory – which is just as well, otherwise we would become irrevocably sensitised to each and every food we consumed, and would only be able to eat them once. IgA is very thymus dependent, and gives rise to the most common of the immunodeficiencies, affecting about one in 700 people. These individuals tend to suffer a higher risk of sinopulmonary and gastrointestinal infections and a greater incidence of food sensitivities.

Hypoallergenic foods
People in this country are very rarely allergic to sago (from the trunk of a palm tree). Similarly, tapioca is usually safe; it is only 2 per cent protein and is derived from African cassava. There have been no reported cases of allergy to rhubarb.

ELIMINATION DIET

If you suspect a food, leave it out of the diet completely for a week. You have to be very strict about this; cutting down is suffering for nothing. If you suspect a sensitivity and wish to test for it, it is all or nothing at all. It also means that all canned or processed and packeted foods are out for that week, because you are never absolutely sure what is in them. If you are eliminating wheat, this means eliminating everything that may contain even a trace of wheat. It probably even means not baking with wheat for the rest of the family, as you would be likely to get some wheat this way. Similarly, it is no use using wheat flour to roll out your oatcakes if you are testing for wheat sensitivity.

If you are addicted to the food you are eliminating, withdrawal symptoms will probably occur during the first three days. Sometimes these can be very violent. If this happens, it may be necessary to come off the food slowly before withdrawing it completely. If you are really this hooked, medical help may be needed in order to give it up. For most people, though, symptoms are unpleasant, but mild and bearable, and usually disappear by the fourth day.

Leave the food out of the diet for the rest of the week or perhaps longer. Then pick a convenient day, if there is such a thing, when it does not matter if you do not perform your best and reintroduce the offending food or beverage on an empty stomach. If there are no violent symptoms, take it several more times throughout the day – in fact, make a pig of yourself on it. If you are allergic to it you should start to feel ill!

It may be necessary to eliminate foods that cause a reaction for six months or so; if this is the case, it will be necessary to find other foods to provide the nutrients that would have been supplied. After a period of time, the food may be reintroduced into the diet, and if it does not then cause any ill effect you can have it occasionally, but never again on a daily basis.

ROTATION DIET

We could all do with a diet where all real foods are eaten in moderation and in rotation, but this is not easy. We all get into our little daily habits.

The best plan of action for people with multi-allergies is to separate the food groups, eating, for example, wheat on Monday, oats and no wheat at all on Tuesday, rice for Wednesday, and so on. Some experts say that a four-day rotation diet will do: others say a seven-day rotation is necessary. It is probably safer and easier to go for the seven-day rotation, the idea being that any offending food is totally eliminated for six days. This six-day gap does not allow the body to build up an addiction to the food and, most importantly, it allows you to eat! If wheat causes aggravation, for example, it is possible to leave it out for several months as long as it is replaced by another grain. (Most people in Britain live on a restricted diet of only one or two grains anyway.) Be adventurous, give your immune system a treat and vary your grains (see Chaper 17).

UNSUCCESSFUL SLIMMING

Dr Berger is a doctor, a psychiatrist and a specialist in bariatrics (the science of weight control). He himself was once an enormous 30 stone (420 lb or 190 kg) and could not lose weight. He tried all of the methods then used for weight loss, but they only made him sicker. He delved into nutritional immunology and found a secret that worked for him and one that has apparently worked for more than 3,000 of his patients who between them lost 74,000 lb (34,000 kg) of extra fat.

He is of the opinion that food sensitivities prevent many people from losing weight. He therefore recommends detection and elimination or rotation of problem foods. After the sensitivities have been identified, supplements help to repair the damaged immune system and allow stored fat to be utilised properly. The best way to slim is slowly, as this way the skin and stomach gradually go back to their normal size and do not look baggy. Sudden shock weight-loss can lead to severe immune deficiency and can eventually perpetuate the fat cycle; in short, inappropriate dieting can make you fat.

HINTS FOR PEOPLE WITH FOOD SENSITIVITIES

- Reduce the number of antigens if possible; that is to say, eliminate chemicals and, as far as possible, the foods to which you are very sensitive. At the same time be careful not to put the diet out of balance. (The book *Allergies: Your Hidden Enemy* will be useful.)
- Improve protein digestion by chewing food well and eating it separate from carbohydrates. In this way, whole proteins are less likely to pass through the gut wall into the body. (*Food Combining for Health* will help with this type of eating pattern.)
- Improve gut mucosal integrity with nutrients, in particular, zinc, pantothenic acid and beta-carotene.
- Reduce sugar and spices which aggravate gut membranes.
- Reduce animal fat consumption and increase the intake of linoleic acid.
- Increase the intake of antioxidants – vitamins E and C, beta-carotene, zinc, copper and manganese.

CONCLUSION

Food sensitivities, as we have seen, cause a vast range of physical, mental and emotional problems. Some people become addicted or develop eating disorders like bingeing, because the foods which cause the damage release beta-endorphins. These are brain chemicals that act a bit like opium; they give relief from pain and give a sensation of well-being; they control appetite, sexual desire and body temperature; but eventually they cause depression. Food can give us pleasure or cause us pain; it can make us fit or make us sick. There is a very strong link between our nutrition and the immune system.

Food allergy is not a simple disease. It is a condition of many causes, many mechanisms and no single cure.

It must be remembered that most people do not have serious food allergies and most people should be able to eat and enjoy a wide variety of foods.

13
THE NUTRITION CONNECTION

How often have you heard 'If you eat a good balanced diet you'll be fine.' Unfortunately, no one ever spells out this enigmatic diet – it's, well, you know, a little bit of everything.

In our search for, or ignorance of, this good, balanced diet, we can tip the scales one way or the other and one of three conditions can result – under-nutrition, malnutrition or over-nutrition – all of which can lead to imbalances in the immune system.

UNDER-NUTRITION

We tend to link problems of under-nutrition with the poorer countries where they do not have enough food, due to drought, famine, overpopulation or simply a lack of knowledge and resources for growing foods which would provide a balanced diet. We see sad pictures of starvation and often hear of epidemics associated with these conditions, because the immune systems of these people are too weak to put up a fight. Starvation, in this context, is simply lack of food, especially protein and usually fat and micronutrients too. The calorie intake is just not sufficient to provide the building blocks necessary to maintain and repair the body, let alone to provide energy and fight disease.

Every day more than half of the world's population goes to bed hungry because they do not have enough food. We do not realise this because, living in the affluent west, we have probably never felt really hungry. Peckish, yes, or the 'It's lunchtime feeling', but not really hungry.

In many areas of the world, the main meal is nearly always a bowl of rice. In Brazil, there may be more variety – perhaps beans, corn and rice – but still a meal deficient in many of the nutrients needed to sustain long healthy life. In Brazil the average amount of meat eaten per person per day is 70 grams, but they are lucky; people in India average around 4 grams, and only eight eggs per person per year. In the west we eat nearly 300 grams of meat per day on average.

Marasmus and kwashiorkor are the two most common conditions. Marasmus is the starvation of babies and usually occurs in poorer countries because mothers stop breastfeeding too early and put them on formula feeds which are often made up incorrectly or under dirty conditions.

Kwashiorkor means first-second in the language of the Ga tribe from Ghana, where the illness is common. It was so named because it is often caused by a second baby feeding at the breast whilst the first is removed too soon and weaned on to a protein-deficient gruel. It is very common in poor countries where religion, ignorance or poverty mean that children are deprived of eggs, milk, fish or meat and live almost entirely on carbohydrate diets. A child on a protein-deficient diet will have stunted growth, will lack energy and will be anorexic, with watery diarrhoea. Oedema often hides muscle wasting, but the liver becomes very fatty and all the other organs become abnormal. It is remarkable that almost all of the symptoms are reversible given the simple medicine of protein-sufficient food.

Under-nutrition can, however, occur in this country, especially amongst abused children, people on ill-advised slimming diets, and lonely or depressed elderly people. Telltale signs, apart from loss of weight, are famine oedema (swelling due to water leakage and accumulation in connective tissue, and loss of elasticity in the tissue), reduced physical activity, dry skin with brown patches, peripheral cyanosis (i.e. fingers, toes, nose, etc., turning blue), slow pulse, irritability, apathy and disorientation. Infections of any kind are common, as the immune system is weak, leaving the body open to attack by any bug that happens to be around.

When food intake drops below maintenance level, the body draws on its own energy reserves which are mainly the triglycerides in our adipose tissue or, in plain English, our fat. In this country healthy men are around 12 per cent fat and healthy women 26 per cent fat, but fat stores of relatively healthy people in places like Bangladesh are much lower. The optimum level is somewhere in between, probably lower than ours but nowhere near as low as theirs.

Once 25 per cent of our natural (not excess) body fat has been lost, death is a possibility, though anything up to 50 per cent has been recorded. Wasting of all tissue, except the brain, will occur and the heart can shrink to as little as a third of its normal weight. The small intestine becomes thinner and thinner until it is practically transparent; in this condition, it loses the ability to absorb nutrients properly.

MALNUTRITION

Although we associate this with TV pictures of starvation, it really means bad nutrition (*mal* being the French adjective for wrong or bad). A lot of people suffer from this condition although they often do not recognise it as such.

In this day and age we eat food either out of habit or for pleasure, with little regard as to why we are doing it and what we actually need. How often, for example, do you get up in the morning and choose a breakfast high in vitamin B$_2$ because your eyes are itchy, or with zinc in it because you have noticed white spots in your nails, or with high beta-carotene levels because you have mouth ulcers? Not often, I suspect. Most people fall into their usual habit of tea or coffee whilst they reach for toast or their favourite cereal.

The real reason for eating should be to give your body the building blocks it needs to build, maintain and repair a good long-lasting healthy, happy and active model.

OVER-NUTRITION

This is probably the most common disease in the western world, and unfortunately, usually refers to an over-consumption of calories, rather than over-supply of a wide range of essential nutrients. It seems that at any given moment (but especially before Christmas and the summer holiday season, when the figures soar) at least 50 per cent of the population wish they were slimmer.

The reasons for over-eating are many and contradictory. For example, some people over-eat because they enjoy the social life that revolves around eating; they eat because they are happy doing so. Others eat because they are unhappy, as though they can fill up the emotional void with food. Some people will eat to lessen the pain of bereavement (although others will totally reject food after this sort of experience and become overly thin). Many will eat because they face exams or have a sedentary job.

Another group of people eat because they always seem to feel hungry; they crave food, possibly because the food they eat is refined, low in the essential micronutrients necessary for health. Their bodies keep passing them the message that they need more micronutrients, and hence more food, even though it is already filled up with devitalised rubbish.

Whatever the reason for over-eating, the result is almost certainly increased body weight, and this can lead to obesity.

Obesity

The ability to store fat in adipose tissue was a necessary adaptation for animals who left the sea, where there was an abundant and constant source of food. Phylogenetically, the arthropods (a group of animals containing not only crustaceans, like crabs and lobsters, but also the insects and spiders) were the first to do this and later birds and mammals developed the principle further. Storing fat in compact form throughout the body was originally an advantage, improving the chances of survival if food became scarce, but it has become a handicap in today's affluent societies where under-activity, together with over-nutrition, have upset the delicate supply and demand balance. We now have an obesity epidemic, together with all its associated diseases.

Obesity is merely excess adipose tissue (fat stores), excess meaning roughly anything over 10 per cent of the norm for any given person. Statistics show that 30 per cent of men and 40 per cent of women are 20 lb (9 kg) or more overweight. Men usually deposit this extra weight on their chest and waistline, whilst women deposit it on their hips, thighs and upper arms.

There are anatomically two distinct types of obese persons:

- Those with an increased number of adipose cells, indicating overfeeding in childhood or between the ages of 9 and 13 (children's food is considered on pages 105–7).
- Those with adult onset obesity, which is characterised by a normal number of adipose cells of increased size.

There are behavioural differences in the two groups, the former suffering much more from depression, fatigue and anxiety; slimming is also less likely to be so effective with this group of individuals.

Fat and the immune system

Carrying a lot of excess fat can stress the heart, the lungs, the liver and the kidneys. It plays havoc with your hormones, increases the risk of cancer or diabetes and lowers resistance to infectious diseases.

Too much fat in the diet can also slow down the immune system considerably, as the fatty acids are absorbed straight from the gut into the lymphatic system, unlike amino acids and sugars, which go into the bloodstream. A lot of fat going into the lymph can make it very heavy to push around, and it also makes it easier for bacteria to hide and escape your immune army.

HOW TO LOSE WEIGHT

If you are lucky and your weight problem is merely one of overeating, restricting your calories whilst eating a sensible varied diet should do the trick. But it is often not that simple and not fast enough, so the temptation is to resort to very restricted fad diets, appetite suppressants or artificial cocktails instead of meals. Unfortunately, in the long run, these methods could even make you fatter and may well cause you to become deficient in many of the micronutrients. These regimes should definitely not be followed for long periods of time. Many people have found that they have ended up fatter, with more health problems, after they have resorted to such drastic dieting methods. It may not happen to you, but why chance it? If a job is worth doing, it is worth doing properly. And, after all, being slim is only part of the carrot; you also expect good health and vitality, not constant headaches, loose and sagging pale skin, sunken eyes, extreme fatigue, dizziness and poor concentration.

It is only just being recognised that not only does excess weight slow down the immune system, but that the immune system has several effects on our ability to maintain normal body weight. As the fat piles on, the immune system becomes less efficient and therefore has less control over body weight, so the problem becomes self perpetuating.

The immune system has a regulatory effect on the digestion, absorption and storage of food. It also determines how effectively we convert our nutrients into energy. Even weight loss itself, i.e. the burning up of fat, is dependent on the state of the immune system and upon having sufficient of the nutrients necessary for carrying out chemical reactions that turn fat into heat or energy.

The best way to lose weight is to do it slowly, sensibly and safely. You have to acknowledge the fact that the fat has built up or been there for a number of years and that the body has to a limited extent become used to it. To stop eating suddenly or to eat only grapes or artificial powders could easily put your biochemistry into a tailspin.

There is no one simple way for everyone to lose weight – we are all different. But there are a few secrets to losing weight, staying that way and remaining healthy into the bargain.

THE SECRETS OF SENSIBLE SLIMMING

- Get yourself as fit as possible (considering your excess weight), first by boosting your immune system, with supplements initially, so that you have all the micro-nutrients necessary to use up that excess fat; and by giving up all junk food and getting on to a healthy diet of whole unrefined foods.
- Mentally prepare yourself as well; if possible slim with someone, and tell your family and friends. That way you are more likely to stick to your plan.
- Set aside a preparation time and a list of snack foods, e.g. cooked rice or carrots, already scraped in a box in the fridge, for those moments when you just have to have a nibble.
- Set yourself a sensible calorie limit (not below 1000). Spread these out through the day, choosing high-nutrient low-calorie whole foods. Small frequent meals are better than one big one as the latter stretches the stomach and keeps it large; small meals allow it to shrink.
- At least half of your food should be complex carbohydrate, in the form of vegetables and grains. There are many other grains besides wheat – try some. (Many diets stress restriction of carbohydrate, because it does give a quick easy fall in weight. Unfortunately, this is mainly due to associated diuresis and there is usually slow progression after the initial loss, because the body adapts to lower energy intake.)
- Restrict foods that are more than 20 per cent fat by weight. No more than one-third of the calories should come from fat. Fat should not be totally polyunsaturated, neither should it be entirely saturated, but it must include the essential fatty acids (see Chapter 14), especially cold-pressed linoleic acid, which is essential for weight loss. Women especially need this if they are to lose weight without losing too much from the breast.
- Slimming children need more protein in relation to body weight than adults.
- Eat only when hungry.
- Avoid the use of all artificial colours and flavours, and keep salt to an absolute minimum.

- The herbs used when slimming are very important for maintaining and enjoying the treatment:

  H is for humour, which is an essential for keeping you in balance. Some slimmers get very serious and intense; they can also become depressed and moody. So do not leave humour on the top shelf.

  E is for encouragement, which you must remind everyone to give you; enthusiasm, which you have to generate yourself; and exercise, which is absolutely essential, because it makes you feel good, gives you something to grumble about and makes you feel that you have done something positive about losing weight during the day. Choosing the right exercises for you helps to keep your body in the right proportion.

  R is for relaxation, to balance the stress and all that exercise, as well as right thinking to maintain your positive state of mind.

  B is for the all-important balance. This is the key to health, but very difficult to attain. It is the right physical, mental and emotional balance, as well as the right balance of food, which makes for any healthy body and personality.

  S is for sociability (people need people, especially when they are trying to achieve a goal); and for supplements, to get the micronutrients right for burning up the fat. The B vitamins and various minerals are necessary for the efficient completion of the fat cycle; if they are deficient, fat cannot be used up properly.

- One of the least recognised causes for overweight is food sensitivity. It is very unfortunate if this is the reason for your excess weight, because we are usually sensitive to the foods that we enjoy the most and crave; so it can be difficult to give them up (see Chapter 12).

- Finally, never go shopping on an empty stomach or you will fill your trolley up with all the sweets, pastries, cakes and biscuity-type foods that you are thinking about. Shop after a meal and you will think clearly about the foods which you should be eating and will not crave for pies and sweets – and you will probably spend less. The trouble is that you always tend to think about food shopping when you are hungry.

STARTING A FAMILY

The importance of good nutrition in childhood is often missed, but the building blocks laid down at this time, and even before birth, form the pattern for health in later life.

It is important for both parents to have adequate zinc, especially if they hope for a boy; all-girl families often have zinc-deficient parents. Pumpkin seeds should become a staple part of the diet at this time, as they are rich in zinc.

Linoleic acid is an essential in the mother's diet, to ensure immune development of the baby and for production of adequate breastmilk afterwards.

Folic acid, choline, vitamin B_{12} and methionine have been shown to be essential for the development of the immune system of the unborn child. The immune organs, especially the thymus, of babies whose mothers were sufficient in these nutrients, were larger and the immune system stronger than those whose mothers were deficient. So fish, eggs, and foods containing B vitamins are very important during pregnancy.

BABIES

There are many reasons for the superiority of breastmilk over other milks for feeding babies. It is, after all, the food intended for baby humans, providing nutrients in the required amounts for the correct development of a baby. No other formula is quite like breastmilk. Breastfed babies are less likely to be overweight than those on artificial feeds.

One of the main advantages of breastmilk is that it, and particularly colostrum, are very high in IgA antibodies. The IgA precursors arising in the Peyer's patches of the mother's intestine home in on the mammary tissue during lactation. There is a special piece of immunoglobulin molecule which goes with each IgA molecule and protects it from digestion in the baby's gut, just as it does in the adult gut. This IgA protects the baby from bacterial, viral and even food antigens. The infant who is artificially fed is exposed to foreign milk proteins at a time when he is unable to produce his own IgA.

Decades ago, child mortality was high because of infections and malnourished mothers. At that time, weight increase in a baby was very important and meant survival. Nowadays, few babies die for these reasons, but we still cling to increased birth weight as a sort of recognition that you are doing all right as a mother. Weight gain is important, but it is not a race to see whose baby puts on most weight each week. Too much is not always better. Formula feeds should never be made up stronger than the recommendations. The water content is as important as the solid content; immature kidneys could have problems if feeds are too concentrated. Remember a baby is more susceptible to infections than an older child, so, boil and cool any liquid to be given.

I am not a fan of soya milk for babies, as it is very low in methionine which is essential for the maturing immune system. Equally, sugared juices are not really advisable for babies; babies are quite happy with water if they are thirsty. Gripe water is high in sugar as well as alcohol; if you take body weight into account, one swig of gripe water has the equivalent effect on a baby to a quarter pint of lager on an adult. The body needs zinc to make the necessary liver enzyme, alcohol dehydrogenase, to detoxify this alcohol, and a baby's diet is usually low in zinc; furthermore, the mother is often zinc deficient and so are formula feeds. Gripe water is therefore not a good idea on a regular basis.

Eczema

Sometimes, but not always, eczema is caused by a lack of linoleic acid; this type of eczema occurs more often when the mother has been avoiding fat during pregnancy to keep her weight down. Linoleic acid, remember, is one of the three essential fatty acids. So if on a low-fat diet during pregnancy, it is worth taking half a teaspoon of cold-pressed safflower oil daily.

This type of eczema is often cleared by giving the baby a very small amount of this oil (only about one-eighth of a teaspoon) every day.

Weaning

A lot of unnecessary fuss is made about weaning. Many, especially first-time, mothers feel that they cannot possibly give babies the nutrients which they need, so they buy packets or tins which they feel have been produced by somebody who knows. However, a baby is far more likely to get the required nutrients from fresh cooked rather than processed food, unless, of course, mum and dad live on junk food. Egg, fish, cheese or meat along with milk and water plus liberal amounts of fresh fruit and vegetables are nutritious real foods, as are the cereal products like rice, oats, millet, semolina or barley. Leave out the salt and sugar. Note that Marmite is 10 per cent salt and should not be used for babies, while the sugar content of rusks is higher than that of a doughnut, so rusks should not become a staple part of the diet. Bran is a refined food and should not be added to a baby's food; it is much too irritating by itself for an immature gut.

Do not wean too early and only introduce one new food at a time. Egg is a good starter, as the baby's iron reserves will be getting low at around six months; eggs are also a good source of methionine, which is essential for the developing immune system. Rice is a good starter and better than wheat to begin with as it does not contain gluten, which can sometimes cause problems; it is about a quarter of the cost of baby rice if you buy whole-grain rice and cook, sieve or liquidise it yourself or grind it in a coffee grinder first. This cheaper rice provides far more nutrients than the white flaked baby rice, so why pay more for less?

Mashed vegetables and mashed fruit are very acceptable dishes, perhaps thinned down a little with milk, water or fruit juice to start with, but do not stew baby's fruit in aluminium pans as immature kidneys are not good at getting rid of this metal. Preferably, do not use aluminium pans at all; use stainless steel or glass.

Artificial colours, sweeteners and flavour enhancers are banned from baby foods for good reason, so do not be lulled into an 'anything goes attitude' and give your baby soft drinks and popular snacks containing these additives.

The immune system in a baby's gut is learning. Breastmilk is best, water is essential. Real, unrefined foods, high in nutrients should be given when he is ready. Refined foods, low in nutrients but high in calories, will only put on weight, not health. Remember, a baby needs the other immune boosters like natural light, fresh air, movement and touch, as well as the right balance of light and dark, sound and silence, stimulation and sleep. Have a happy, healthy baby.

TODDLERS AND YOUNG CHILDREN

Toddlers should be encouraged right away to eat good food. I have little time for a mother who says that her child will only eat fish fingers or sausages and chips at meal times and who screams if she does not get her sweets.

Similarly, I have not much sympathy for those who say 'Well, I haven't time to do breakfast. I haven't time to make a proper packed lunch.' 'At tea time my child is so hungry that she needs something right away.' 'I haven't time to prepare it.' Having babies is a responsibility and parents should make time to feed their children properly.

In relation to body weight, a growing child needs more protein than an adult. She has a body to build. She is still more susceptible to illness than an adult as she has not yet had time to build up a memory bank of antibodies. Chocolate bars, crisps, sweets and soft drinks just do not provide anywhere near enough of the necessary nutrients – just calories.

Popular children's food

Take fish fingers, sausages and burgers. These are classic ways of turning cheap ingredients into highly flavoured low-nutrient food for children.

Fish fingers are no longer pieces of fish in breadcrumbs. The fish can be as little as a third of the weight of the finger. They are thus really very expensive forms of fish. To add insult to injury, the fish is not prime flesh but scrappy poor-grade reconstituted mince that a proud pet owner would be unlikely to feed to her prize cat.

A sausage too is padded out so that manufacturers can sell water, rusk, additives and fillers instead of meat. How much it is disguised can be seen by the degree of shrinking and the amount of liquid which comes out on cooking. It is another small protein package and, although it may be a cheap stomach filler, it is usually very expensive for the nutrients it offers.

Burgers are similar. You may be lucky and know a butcher who makes his burgers with good fresh meat, but the chances are you will be tucking into flavoured and textured minced skin, feet, head, tail and gristle. Again, the low-nutrient burgers fill and satisfy. They taste good, thanks to all the added flavours. They look good, compliments of the added colour. They feel good, due to added emulsifiers and stabilisers. They keep a long time and are easy to prepare, courtesy of the added preservatives. But how much of this chemical concoction can your system use to build a healthy body with? How much hinders the normal working of a healthy immune system?

Food pellets are no longer just for animals. We now feed them to children. Corn starch or potato starch, well refined and treated to last indefinitely, is mixed up, blobbed into pretty shapes, fried and covered with all sorts of chemical wonders to make them taste and look exciting. The nutritional value of these snack pellets is hard to define; the chemical burden is easier to calculate. Like crisps, these snacks are around 40 per cent fat and are usually high in salt and other chemicals.

Children need real food that will make bodies which will last. These fast foods are all right occasionally, but not as a stable part of the diet. Food additives, especially dyes contained in many of these dead foods, cause problems such as hyperactivity, bedwetting and other behavioural disorders. Orange and yellow dyes used in squashes, lollies, fish fingers, batters and other such foods are very likely to cause frequent and sometimes involuntary urination; frequency returns to normal on removal of these dyes. Playschools can help here by encouraging children to bring or have fruit, vegetables and wholefood snacks with milk or fruit juice for the morning break.

Young children on a good diet do not usually need supplements other than vitamin C as their absorption of nutrients is good. However, some children on inadequate diets do need extra. It is best to consult a professional for individual guidance if there are any special problems, e.g. vitamin C (500 mg per day) helps prevent tooth decay and wards off infections. If a child starts a cold this dosage can be increased, but is best spread out in small amounts throughout the day and taken with plenty of fluid. A suckable zinc supplement is also a good idea.

A child may voluntarily miss food for a day if she is feeling ill. This is acceptable, as long as she drinks plenty of fluids, but certainly no child should be compelled to fast or be put on any restricted diet unless for medical reasons and under medical supervision. Asthmatics should not be encouraged to eat polyunsaturated fats all the time, as these spreads often make their condition worse.

Children who only eat processed foods have a very restricted diet and would need food supplements, however it would be better to improve their diet.

CHILDHOOD TO ADOLESCENCE

This is a notorious time for behaviour problems. This is hardly surprising as there are a lot of chemical changes going on in the body, in particular the turning up of sex hormone production and the turning down of the immune system. It is a time of great change, mentally, physically, emotionally and immunologically.

Growth hormone stimulates the immune system, whilst sex hormones depress it. The immune system is the first of all of our bodily systems to show signs of aging, and this process starts at puberty. All these quite drastic chemical, physical and emotional changes are rather like having to change gear in a car fairly fast and frequently. For the inexperienced driver, as all teenagers are, this can make for a very bumpy ride, but matters are often made worse by the inappropriate fuel they use.

Diet

The Department of Health reckons that the average teenager needs about 75 grams of protein per day. As I stand in the dinner queue at school, watching the ever-popular beans and chips plates disappear, often even without the token burger or fish finger, I have to wonder where the teenagers get their nutrients from – home, I hope. I know however that many of them skip breakfast and others have high-calorie, sugar-laden, low-nutrient, breakfast cereal and that most of them eat crisps and chocolate bars every day.

The average 2-ounce burger has only 12 grams of protein, and the fish in a fish finger need only be one-third of that finger, the rest being filler, while the fish content of a fishcake may be even less. Because of this many teenagers in an affluent country such as ours may well be marginally deficient in protein. This does not show itself as an obvious illness, but it may show up in other ways: they cannot hold themselves up straight; they constantly slouch or hold their heads up with their hands; and, perhaps most significantly, they cannot mount an effective immune response to infection.

No matter what living thing you are dealing with, it will have certain specific requirements which must be met before it can live properly. A growing developing body has many requirements. Nutrients are only a part of these requirements, but they are a vital part; not too much and not too little of each are required. Appetite should control our needs, but we trick it by refining vital nutrients out of our food. Satisfying our hunger does not necessarily mean we satisfy our nutrient needs if we eat only devitalised food. Vitamins, minerals and accessory food factors are also vital to health. Living off single-nutrient foods like sugar and virtually nutrient-free junk like some soft drinks will not build healthy resistant long-lasting bodies.

Many of our children and teenagers eat high-energy foods, that is the simple carbohydrates that are intended to give the body energy. Yet are they energetic? Not a bit of it. Many drag themselves around, or prop themselves up in front of the television set. Repeated research from Strathclyde and Exeter Universities shows that teenage girls, in particular, are very sedentary. The instant energy provided by a refined carbohydrate snack cannot be used instantly if the nutrients needed for its metabolism are not present. Instead the energy is lost in a transient high mood followed by a long low, most of the sugar getting converted to saturated fat and then stored. It seems that when essential fatty acids, in particular, are insufficiently supplied, a body changes sugar into fat much more rapidly than would be expected under sufficient conditions. It is as though the body were trying to make up for the missing nutrients. Unfortunately, though, the essential ones cannot be made by the body. This leads to a vicious circle of more sugar being required to keep up with this altered metabolism.

The more sugar is eaten, the more insulin has to be produced, but insulin is one of the hormones which encourages the body to store fat, along with cortisol and the three sex hormones (teenagers get an increase in these too).

Controversy rages about breakfast – eat it, do not eat it, eat fruit only, etc. Repeatedly, reliable research has shown that the best way to maintain blood sugar levels, without having any artificial highs and lows which cause the mood swings, fits of energy or lethargy and poor concentration, is to start the day with protein and complex carbohydrate. I think this is important for young people; the ups and downs of body chemicals are enough to cope with at that age without a blood-sugar seesaw as well. The trouble is that many teenagers, girls in particular, do not feel like having breakfast. The meal need not be large, however, but should include egg, milk, yoghourt or fish, and some complex carbohydrate such as bread or a wholegrain cereal (Weetabix, Shredded Wheat, oats, muesli, etc.). If the individual really cannot eat a lot, half an egg, a quarter of a piece of wholemeal bread or toast and a cup of milk is better at keeping an even keel than a bowl of refined sugared cereal and squash or just coffee. Eat as much or as little as desired at breakfast, but eat unrefined carbohydrate and protein. (If any of the family follow the Hay diet, which necessitates the separation of concentrated proteins and carbohydrates, this combination can be achieved using fruit and yoghourt.)

Fibre, fruit and vegetables are obviously essential, but fish should also be an important inclusion in the diet, preferably at least twice a week. It offers protection from heart disease as well as supplying those essential fats, proteins and minerals needed for the immune system. Cartilaginous fish, like skate and shark, do not have bone problems, although teenagers really ought to be capable of boning a mackerel, plaice or cod. Fish oils can be supplemented, if necessary, but the real thing is a better choice. The other group of essential fats are also important for teenagers (see Chapter 14); they should be included as a supplement if not part of the regular diet.

Food supplements may be necessary, but again it is better to have these worked out by a professional who will take individual dietary likes and dislikes as well as lifestyle and special needs into consideration. Zinc, however, warrants special mention, being vital for the immune system, sex development and enzyme systems. Many teenagers are short of this mineral as it is low in our soil and is refined out of many foods. A deficiency shows itself as white spots in the nails and/or spots on the skin – 15 mg of zinc citrate daily for a few weeks should correct this. New white spots should not appear, but the old ones in the nails will have to grow out. Spots on the skin may improve drastically if they are due to zinc deficiency.

B vitamins may also be very useful around period time for girls, and exam time; they need only be taken when needed (50 mg B complex). Because man has lost his ability to make vitamin C, this is always a useful supplement to have as a powder in the cupboard, to be used at the first sign of an infection. It lessens discomfort, hastens recovery and may even prevent the infection or cold completely if you manage to get the dose right and take it fast enough.

A final note on the much maligned chip. Everyone seems to think that nutritionists are against chips, whereas, in reality, most of us rate them as quite good food if they are cooked properly and not eaten exclusively. They need only be around 10 per cent fat, which is good in comparison to crisps which are 40 per cent fat. (Low-fat varieties of crisps are not much better than the ordinary ones as some of the fat is replaced with glucose syrup – hardly a healthy alternative.) So what makes a healthy chip?

- A thick-cut or scalloped chip is less fattening. Thin chips soak up much more fat than fat ones.
- Potatoes that have been parboiled or soaked in water, preservative or stuff that prevents discolouring allow greater fat uptake. Freshly cut ones are better.
- Chips should be cooked in fresh polyunsaturated oil or lard, not in reheated or stale fat. Many health professionals will disagree with me on lard, but I think it is a good fat to cook with as it does not carry the increased cancer risk factor that heated, and especially reheated, polyunsaturates do. It does not carry a heart disease risk either, unless the total fat intake is excessive or unbalanced. It is roughly half saturated and half monounsaturated fat (see page 114).
- Chips need to be well drained and excess fat wiped off.
- Chips are healthier served without salt, and not at every meal.
- They are also good chipped with their skins on.

Conclusion

There are many factors that all work together to make a teenager happy and healthy – and I am by no means discounting emotional, social, genetic and all the other factors which are involved in this, but I think that we could considerably improve the behaviour, performance, concentration, learning ability and health of our young people by making their diet nutritionally adequate and encouraging them to take more exercise.

14
FATS

Just as every individual has their own fingerprints, they also have their own chemical composition, although, unlike their fingerprints, it is constantly changing. If we generalise, we are over 70 per cent water, added to which are a handful of chemicals – and the rest is a rancidifying lump of fat. What a romantic thought!

WHAT IS FAT?

Fats are made up of carbon, hydrogen and oxygen. The correct term for all the naturally occurring fat-like substances is lipid. The triglycerides in the blood and the common fats and oils that we eat are simple lipids. The phospholipids are compound lipids and are important in our body chemistry, but we are probably less familiar with them; they are very important for cell wall membranes, for metabolism of fat in general and as a component of brain and nervous tissue. The best known phospholipid is phosphatidylcholine (lecithin); an enzyme which attacks lecithin is the active ingredient of the venoms of many snakes and poisonous insects. Steroids are usually grouped with the lipids and include bile acids, sex and adrenal hormones and cholesterol.

HOW MUCH FAT?

In Britain it is estimated that we eat on average 4½ ounces (125 grams) of fat per day, although the recommendation is to bring this down to 100 grams a day. Fats are about twice as high in calories as proteins or carbohydrates and make up 38 to 40 per cent of our total calorie intake. This is really much too high. People in third world countries consume far less than 20 per cent, but they are at the other extreme. The ideal fat content of our diet is probably somewhere between 25 and 30 per cent of our calorie intake. Fat intake, however, should not be dropped suddenly. It should be decreased gradually over a period of time.

Most people neither have the time nor the inclination to count the calories they eat, work out the fat content and turn it into percentages. So it is easier to use a rough guide. Those foods that are less than 20 per cent fat (by weight, not calories) can be used as part of the everyday diet without too much concern. Those that are above this level need a lot more thought as to balance and quantity; for example, crisps, chocolate bars and sausages should not be staples of our diet, although, unfortunately, they are becoming so for many of our children. These foods are all high in calories, high in fat, high in salt or sugar and low in nutrients – just the ingredients for a short unhealthy life. There is no reason, however, why they cannot be enjoyed occasionally.

WHY EAT FAT AT ALL?

Even if we eat no fat, we will make it from excess carbohydrates and proteins; for example, the latter can be converted into fat if we eat more than we need for growth, repair and topping up our amino acid pool. The body cannot, however, make the essential fatty acids, and these have to be supplied in the diet to maintain health and normal body weight.

The body needs fat – for padding and shape, and to protect bones, nerves, blood vessels and internal organs. It is also needed as insulation, in order to maintain a constant body temperature, and for immediate as well as stored energy. However its use as a reserve food, i.e. as a long-term energy reserve, is rarely needed in this country.

In order for fat to be both built up and broken down properly, other nutrients are required, in particular linoleic acid (itself an essential fat), the B group of vitamins, especially choline and inositol, and magnesium. Without sufficient of these extra substances, it may be very difficult either to put weight on (if you are too thin), to take weight off (if you are too fat) or to metabolise and store fat properly. One study which fed starving dogs pig fat found that the dogs stored the fat that they ate, but had not managed to convert it into dog fat because they did not have the nutrients to do this. There is the possibility that people who store ugly fat that does not fit the body are not converting their fat properly and similarly find it difficult getting rid of it.

In digestion, we break fats down into their building blocks and then use these blocks to build up what we need again. Our efficiency at breaking down and building up fat is crucial to our health and shape, and is nutrient dependent.

ROUGH GUIDE TO FAT

This is a rough guide to the fat content of foods which are, or are often thought to be, high in fat. Be especially aware of those you eat which are in excess of 20 per cent fat by weight; balance their intake with fresh fruit and vegetables.

Oils
Oils are 100 per cent fat.

	Saturated %	Mono-unsaturated %	Poly-unsaturated %
Corn oil	10	30	50
Olive oil	10	75	10
Sunflower oil	10	15	70

Bakery and processed foods

	Fat content %
Chocolate	40
Crisps	40
Pastry	50–33
Biscuits (plain, sweet or crackers)	20
Ice cream (not made with cream)	15
Chips (cut thick)	10
Oats	5
Bread	3

Nuts and seeds
Including legumes that look like nuts.

	Fat content %	
Brazil, pecan, hazelnut	over 60	(mainly polyunsaturated)
Pistachios, peanuts, almonds, beechnuts	50	
Cashews	45	
Sesame seed, sunflower seed	45	
Coconut	35	(almost entirely saturated)

Meat and fish

After removing all visible fat and skin and roasting or grilling in its own remaining fat.

	Fat content %
Bacon, sausages	50
Duck	25
Mackerel & herring	25
Beef, lamb, pork	20
Salmon, turkey	15
Kidney	15
Chicken, veal, tuna	10
Venison, cod	5
Lobster	2
Hake, haddock	1

Fat added during cooking, fatty meat (especially fat hidden in mince) and skin may all put the fat content way above 20 per cent. The above figures apply to lean muscle meat only.

Other fats

	Fat content %	
Lard	100	(half saturated, half mono-unsaturated)
Butter	80	(30 per cent of this is mono-unsaturated)
Margarine	80	(varies a lot depending on brand)
Mayonnaise	80	
Thick cream	40	
Hard cheese	30	
Single cream	20	
Eggs (whole)	12	
Human and goats' milk	4.8	
Cottage cheese	4	
Milk (whole)	3.7	

OBESITY

It is obvious that, under normal circumstances, if we eat too much and move too little, we get fat. If we cut down on food intake and exercise away the fat, and our body chemistry is working fine, we get thinner.

For some people, however, slimming is not as simple as this. They struggle to keep their intake down to a bare 1,000 calories, yet they still remain well padded. Many people have food sensitivities or nutritional deficiencies; some people may well not be eating enough. Too little dietary fat can, ironically, cause you to be overweight, as the body struggles to make the fat it needs from carbohydrates; it cannot, however, make the essential ones which are necessary for regulating fat metabolism – it always has a desire for the fats it needs and so keeps trying to convert more. Sadly, it can never satisfy its real need without the addition of essential fats to the diet. When the body tries to use carbohydrates in the absence of fat, its metabolism speeds up and blood sugar levels go haywire. Cravings for sweets are often experienced, to normalise the blood sugar levels again.

Slimming in the conventional way reduces these people to sick, flabby, lethargic, pale, confused or unhappy patients. They do not look better for weight loss; they look and feel ill.

The carbohydrate-driven person and the waterlogged one often improve and lose weight when linoleic acid is added to the diet. Our diet is very low in untreated linoleic acid; it is best taken as cold-pressed safflower oil, which is the oil highest in linoleic acid.

Low-fat diets

These can be dangerous in themselves. To go quickly from our average 40 per cent to 20 per cent fat intake is not advisable.

One problem with low-fat diets is that the fat soluble nutrients like vitamins A, D, E and K cannot be absorbed in sufficient quantities.

Another is that the gallbladder only empties its bile when fat enters the intestine. In order for the gallbladder to work properly, it must be emptied regularly or it can form stones, go stale and bad, or can even shrink. So do not leave fat out of the diet completely for weeks on end in an attempt to slim – you could ruin your fat digestion for good.

Mineral oils are not fats, they are merely hydrocarbons, made from carbon and hydrogen. They are not food either and should not be used as laxatives or as oil coatings for dried fruit, etc. (They are used for purely cosmetic reasons to stop fruit sticking together; it costs little more to use vegetable oil.) Research shows that over half of any intake of such oils does get into the body via the intestines – it doesn't all pass out with the faeces – and it ties up vitamins A, D, E and K, so causing deficiencies. It is also a possible carcinogen, so avoid both it and any fruit treated with it, or at least wash the oil off with very hot water before eating it.

TYPES OF FAT WE EAT

Saturated fats
Saturated fat is solid at room temperature, and is mainly of animal origin. Coconut and palm fat are the two exceptions; they are cheap and often used in food processing. Coconut fat is almost entirely saturated fat so, per gram of fat, it provides more saturated fat than lard. The product label that boasts 'Containing vegetable fat' may be very saturated indeed if that fat is from coconut.

All saturated fats are good for business, because they are consistent – cakes or biscuits will always taste the same, packet after packet - and have a long shelf life. Chip-shop vegetable fat is often palm or mixed fat.

Mono-unsaturated fats
People of the Mediterranean area eat about 30 per cent of their total calories as fat, but their diet is low in saturated fat. They use a lot of olive oil which is mainly oleic acid, a mono-unsaturated fat.

Mono-unsaturated fats are good to cook with as there is only one double bond which can be broken to give undesirable free radicals, as can be seen in the formula for oleic acid below:

$$CH_3 \cdot (CH_2)_7 \cdot CH=CH(CH_2)_7 \cdot CO_2H$$

Mono-unsaturated fat is reasonably stable and has one free link to transport anything the body wants transported. It does not appear to be linked with any risk of heart disease.

Polyunsaturated fats
Heart disease is a major killer and has been linked to our saturated fat consumption. To try to alter the balance, we have been encouraged to eat more polyunsaturated fat. Unfortunately, we have increased our intake of only one family of polyunsaturates, the n-6 or

omega-6 group. This still leaves us with an unbalanced fat intake (see page 121). Many people are now eating too much of the n-6 polyunsaturates, which may increase the risk of cancer and of different forms of heart and circulatory disorders, such as clots and strokes.

Polyunsaturated fat is needed by the body to transport such things as fat-soluble vitamins. A good way to think of them is to imagine a charm bracelet with a number of double links like the one in oleic acid. One link of these double links can be opened up without breaking the bracelet, and can then be used to hang a charm on or, in this case, a vitamin. As well as vitamins, oxygen or hydrogen can be hung from these double links.

If the fat is exposed to air, and especially when heated, oxygen will be the 'charm' added on to the fatty bracelet. This will cause the fat to go bad and rancid. If hydrogen is added on, instead, then the fat molecules merely become saturated and are only any good as building blocks – they are no longer of any use for transport. A product may well say on the packet that it is made with polyunsaturated fat; what it does not say, is that this fat has been well and truly saturated by exposing it to hydrogen first. This is often done commercially, because the fat keeps longer, but it makes the fat saturated. A clue will be if the label says it contains hydrogenated vegetable fat.

The body can turn some saturated fats into unsaturated fats, i.e remove some of the hydrogen atoms leaving double bonds behind, if it needs free double bonds in order to join various fatty acids together – this is how larger fat molecules can be built up, by linking together fatty acid building blocks via double bonds. To understand this process think again of two chain-link bracelets joined by one free link.

ESSENTIAL FATTY ACIDS

The essential fatty acids have to be provided in the diet because the body cannot make them, because the double bonds are found somewhere in the middle of the chain. Just as we cannot undo a zip from the middle or from the wrong end, so the body cannot unsaturate a fatty acid from any position.

One of the main functions of essential fatty acids is for prostaglandin and leukotriene production, which are necessary for regulating the immune function and blood clotting (see below). They are also needed for hormone production and for feeding our good intestinal bacteria, and are particularly abundant in nervous tissue and the brain.

Every cell is dependent on EFAs in particular for making the cell membrane. With EFA deficiency, cell walls are weaker and more prone to attack by viruses, carcinogens, chemicals or even the body's own immune army. In many auto-immune conditions, correct dosage of EFAs has been shown to be of benefit; for example, a study with MS patients has shown that supplements containing specific EFAs correct abnormal cell membranes, so stabilising the multiple sclerosis. They are also needed for the regulation of fat metabolism and the transport of cholesterol.

There are three important essential fatty acids that the body cannot make out of carbohydrates, protein or saturated fats. These therefore have to be supplied in the diet, and are called linoleic acid, arachidonic acid and alpha-linolenic acid. They are vital for health, weight regulation and immune function.

- Foods rich in linoleic acid are seeds and their natural oils (such as safflower, sunflower, corn, sesame and soybean), nuts, olives, wheat and oatgerm. Chicken and pork have more linoleic acid than lamb, beef or deer, because the bacteria in the rumens of ruminant animals convert the linoleic acid into saturated fat.
- Arachidonic acid (like linoleic acid) belongs to the omega 6 group of fatty acids. It is found in meat and dairy produce, from which we normally get a plentiful supply.
- Alpha-linolenic acid belongs to the omega 3 group of fatty acids and is found in green vegetables, linseed oil, soy oil and phytoplankton. Phytoplankton is the staple diet of many fish, so fish and fish-eating animals also tend to be rich in this EFA.

EFAs and the prostaglandins
All of the essential fatty acids give rise to groups of chemicals known as the prostaglandins. These prostaglandins (or PGs) have various effects in the body:
- The one series of prostaglandins (PG1 series) is involved in the regulation of the T-suppressor lymphocytes and in a decrease in the stickiness, or the ability to clot, of the blood. They therefore decrease the risk of heart disease.
- The two series (PG2), which includes a subgroup called the leukotrienes, are known to increase inflammation and blood clotting. Furthermore, the leukotrienes are involved in asthma and other allergic conditions.
- The three series of prostaglandins (PG3 series), like the PG1s,

reduce the clotting tendency of blood, and are beneficial to anyone with high blood pressure and heart disease.

These three groups of prostaglandins are derived from the three essential fatty acids:

- The PG1 series is derived from linoleic acid.
- The PG2 series is derived from arichidonic acid.
- The PG3 series is derived from alpha-linolenic acid.

It is therefore important to balance the intake of the various essential fatty acids in order to ensure a beneficial balance of the prostaglandins in the body, such that blood clotting and the inflammation response are available at a suitable level when needed, but are not available in excess so that they cannot cause blood clots and inflammation for no reason. For example, a diet rich in mammalian meat tends to produce an overload of the PG2 series and the leukotrienes, which in turn tends to increase the risk of heart disease. A deficiency of the PG1 series also tends to be present in people with auto-immune diseases like rheumatoid arthritis, as well as in those with multiple sclerosis; this is thought to be due to the effect these prostaglandins have on the T suppressor cells. Interestingly, aspirin is often used to treat heart disease and rheumatoid arthritis, and its point of action is at arachidonic acid, preventing the formation of the PG2 series.

FAT BALANCE

The most surprising results are found in traditional Eskimos. They consume a diet very rich in fat – from fish oil and seal fat – but eat their meat raw, so that it contains all of the nutrients necessary for its utilisation. They also eat protective EPA (or eicosapentaenoic acid, which is a derivative of alphalinolenic acid) and their saturated fat is in balance with the unsaturated fat. The PS ratio, the ratio of polyunsaturated to saturated fat in the diet, is the same as for the Eskimo, a poor Indian and a Japanese farmer. The latter two both have very low-fat diets and little heart disease. The Eskimo has a very high-fat diet, but also has little heart disease. All three have a PS ratio of 1 (the PS ratio for an average British diet is 0.2). The amount of fat may not be the important factor in preventing heart disease, if the balance between the types of fat is right. (The amount of fat however is important for other conditions, aging in particular.)

The problem is that, with present trends in factory farming and food processing, we have overdone the saturated fat. A free-living wart hog is less than 5 per cent saturated fat: a pig reared for meat, which has spent its life eating and getting out of breath walking from its shelter to its food trough, is 40 per cent saturated fat.

Eggs from battery hens have much higher levels of saturated fat than eggs from free-range hens, whilst penguin eggs contain mainly unsaturated fat.

Even lard depends on how the pig was fed and exercised, a hard lard being more saturated than a soft one. Lard is usually considered to be half saturated and half mono-unsaturated fat – not the baddie that it is reputed to be.

Food manufacturers obviously try to produce foods that have a reasonably long shelf-life, and saturated fat keeps longer than unsaturated fat so it is used more often.

Our saturated fat consumption is now out of balance with our polyunsaturated fat intake. We have tried to correct this by decreasing the former and increasing the latter, but the polyunsaturates we have used have been those of the omega-6 (n-6) family. There is now concern that our consumption of omega-6 polyunsaturated fatty acids (PUFAs) is too high and is causing problems of its own, increasing the risk of tumour growth, arthritis and thrombosis.

The problem is thus that we do not have enough omega-3 (n-3) PUFAs and we have too much saturated fat and perhaps too much omega-6 PUFAs. Fish oil consumption, along with overall fat reduction, would appear to be a dietary approach to redressing this balance, reducing the risks of cancer, arthritis, thrombosis and of other forms of heart disease caused by an imbalanced fat intake.

Excessive consumption of dietary omega-6 PUFAs are thought to have the following consequences, among others:

- They are thought to alter endocrine (hormone) balance.
- They are thought to stimulate cell division.
- They are thought to alter mammary tissue; in particular, they are thought to be a major contributory factor in breast cancer.
- They are thought to alter immune function.
- They are more prone to forming free radicals, which in turn can damage healthy tissues.
- And, as we have seen, omega-6 stimulate over-synthesis of the 2-series prostaglandins, which are the relatively harmful prostaglandins.

It is possible that the omega-3 PUFAs replace excess omega-6 PUFAs in tumour tissue, so decreasing the prostaglandin production and retarding the growth of tumour cells.

In tumours there are massive invasions of macrophages, which are major producers of prostaglandins. They are usually cytotoxic to tumour cells, but again it is the balance which is crucial. Macrophages which have too many omega-6 PUFAs have too many prostaglandins, and their anti-tumour response is suppressed. Dietary intervention with fish oils may help not only in the prevention of tumours by keeping the fat in balance, but also in treatment, as omega-3 PUFAs increase the production of the enzyme arginase, and it is arginase which is cytolytic to tumours.

CHOLESTEROL

There is a lot of disagreement at present about the role of cholesterol in heart disease. It is true that many people with atherosclerosis (furring up of the arteries, and in particular of those arteries serving the heart itself) have high cholesterol levels in their bloodstream, but is the high cholesterol level the cause of the disease or the result?

One good theory is that blood vessel disease is brought about by free radical or other damage, and that cholesterol is merely attracted to that site of damage, as is calcium. It is possible that the hardened or narrowed blood vessels are caused by calcification and cholesterol build-up, which are the body's attempts at repairing the damage. High cholesterol may be a symptom caused by years of nutrient deficiencies. It is known that cholesterol levels are brought down by the three vitamins, niacin, choline and inositol; by the essential fatty acids, omega-3 PUFAs in particular; and by oat consumption.

We make cholesterol in the body, whatever we eat – we need it to make healthy cell membranes, to make vitamin D, to make the sex and adrenal hormones, and to make bile. A high consumption of saturated fats appears to boost the levels of cholesterol in the bloodsteam; what may be more significant is whether we have enough of the nutrients necessary for cholesterol's utilisation. Animals on diets lacking choline, inositol and essential fatty acids also deposit cholesterol in their arteries, rather like in human atherosclerosis (the furring-up process). High cholesterol problems may be due to insufficient n-3 essential fatty acids and B vitamins rather than just excessive saturated fat intake.

FOOD PROCESSING AND FATS

Once upon a time food was processed at home and you could see just how much fat was eaten. Nowadays we are fortunate in having our food prepared for us, but it often contains fat that we would not suspect was there. Most people would say a bar of chocolate was sugar; yet a bar of chocolate, on average, is 40 per cent fat and 60 per cent sugar. (The simple sugar in this bar, unless followed by quite a lot of exercise, would also be changed into saturated fat in the body.) Crisps, too, are 40 per cent fat, and high in sodium (they are really a way of selling potatoes at an exorbitantly high price). You might think that healthier changes are being made, but things are not always what they seem; for example, when fish and chips and burgers or sausage and chips were labelled high-fat foods, fast food chains jumped on 'healthier chicken' and processed it. Sadly the final product was even higher in fat than the original culprits.

The question of margarine

Margarine is a processed fat. Personally, I neither like nor use margarine. One of the reasons that I do not like it is because of all the labelling dodges, which somehow leave me with the feeling that manufacturers have something to hide. It is also very time consuming to try to decide exactly what it is that you are buying.

- What is a margarine which is low in cholesterol? Vegetable fats do not contain cholesterol in the first place.
- Made with 100 per cent vegetable fat? As I have already mentioned, coconut fat is higher in saturated fat than lard, so where is the advantage?
- Made with 100 per cent sunflower oil? On the back we see the ingredients include hydrogenated vegetable oils, so how much is polyunsaturated sunflower oil?
- Made with polyunsaturated fats? But have they been hydrogenated first and, if not, how did they become solid?

The second main reason for preferring not to use margarine is the amount of processing it may go through. You are not always sure which oil or mixture of oils is used; the oils have to be chemically treated to remove smell, taste and colour, so that the margarine always tastes the same whatever oil mix is used. The mix is then treated again to put back taste and colour; the heat treatment is usually high, but any fat treated above 120°F (50°C) may not be digested properly by pancreatic enzymes. Hydrogenation of unsaturated fats is needed, to some degree, to make the fats solid, otherwise we would have to pour them on to the bread. Hydrogenation produces trans fatty acids; natural ones are cis fatty acids, which are the molecular mirror images of the trans fatty acids. Just like putting the left glove on to the right hand, trans fatty acids do not fit into the body's chemistry and they interfere with the normal metabolism of true essential fatty acids.

WHAT SHOULD WE DO WITH FAT?

- Most people in this country need to reduce their fat intake from the average of 40 per cent down to 30 per cent of the total calorie intake. Again as a rough guide, this is from 125 grams per day to 100 grams per day, but please be sensible about it, not everyone needs to reduce their intake.
- Watch carefully your intake of processed foods which contain hidden fat, and also your intake of foods which are over 20 per cent fat by weight.
- Use of margarine or butter depends on personal choice, but if you prefer butter, eat it. Use willpower to moderate the amount. Use it for bread and butter where you can taste it, but do not bother to put any extra fat on at all if you are eating, say, cheese or baked beans on toast.
- Ensure an adequate intake of omega-6 PUFAs. Personally, I think that margarine is a non-starter and prefer to use cold-pressed natural oils, especially safflower oil. These oils can be used in a salad dressing; they are more beneficial eaten cold – much of the benefit is lost by cooking.
- Ensure sufficient intake of omega-3 PUFAs. These are found in leafy green vegetables, fish and fish oils.
- All oils, but especially the natural untreated ones like cold-pressed oils or cod liver oil, should be stored in an airtight container in the refrigerator.
- When cooking, mono-unsaturated oils like olive oil are probably best as they incur the least risk of heart disease and cancer.
- Polyunsaturated oils may be used once, but re-using them is not a good idea as they pick up oxygen from the air which can increase rancidity and free radical production.
- Lard is a very good stable fat for cooking where olive oil would give an undesirable taste; for example, mushrooms or chips. It is half saturated, half mono-unsaturated, and cheap enough to be able to throw it away often. Butter is also a good fat with which to cook. You cannot overheat it, or it goes brown, unpleasant and you have to throw it away. Like lard, it is stable, and free radical production is much, much less than from the less stable oils.
- Fry only in moderation. Preferably, roast meat in its own fat; do not add any. Grill in preference to frying. Do not have chips or roast potatoes with everything.

- Avoid trans fats as much as possible. These are the chemically altered fats found in processed foods.
- Do not consume mineral oils at all.
- Exercise daily to keep the lymph moving and to use up any surplus sugars which you have eaten so that they are not converted into fat. Remember, fat is absorbed into the lymphatic system and this system has no heart to pump it around – it is dependent on muscular contraction and exercise.
- When you are ill, keep fat intake low; too much clogs up the lymph and slows down your immune army, as well as providing nice fat lumps for bugs to hide behind. Do muscular contraction exercises, even if confined to bed.
- At all times ensure an adequate intake of micronutrients needed to utilise fat, the B vitamins and magnesium in particular.
- Never drastically reduce fat intake; always do it gradually over a period of time and eat some every day to ensure a healthy gallbladder.

15
PROTEINS AND CARBOHYDRATES

If you answer yes to a lot of the questions in the accompanying box, you could be protein deficient. Surprisingly, there are quite a few people who are deficient in protein, even in a country like ours which appears to have ample food. Water retention in pregnancy may well signal protein deficiency, as insufficient albumin may cause a problem with picking up waste water from tissues. People on unbalanced slimming diets, vegans or vegetarians who have just decided to adopt that lifestyle but have not bothered to learn about amino acid combining, fast food addicts, people who live alone and children are most at risk.

PROTEIN DEFICIENCY
- Do you find it difficult to hold yourself up straight when sitting or standing?
- Do you have rounded shoulders, a sunken chest, flat feet?
- Do your hair and nails grow slowly?
- Do you have difficulty concentrating?
- Do you get short periods of depression, anxiety and irritability?
- Is your memory slipping?
- Do you have difficulty sleeping?
- Do you get frequent infections?
- Do you get wandering aches and pains?
- Do you feel that you look older than you are?
- Do you constantly feel hungry?
- Does your mood change frequently?
- Do you have weight problems?
- Do you get indigestion?
- Do you have very low blood pressure?
- Do you suffer from constipation?
- Do you suffer from water retention?

Children and young people need a lot of protein for growth; however, many choose a low-nutrient fast-food diet. Some become vegetarian when their parents are not, and so tend to be given the same meals, but without the meat. Yet others are put on restrictive diets by parents.

WHAT ARE PROTEINS?

Protein is the basic constituent of all living cells. Three-quarters of the dry weight of most body cells is protein. Proteins make up hormones, enzymes, neurotransmitters and antibodies. The name comes from Proteus, a mythological figure who, like protein, could change his form. If we eat cow protein or bean protein, we break it down into its constituent amino acids and then make it up again into the protein we require. The amino acids themselves perform essential functions. Some control depression, memory, sleep, moods, energy levels, relaxation, tension, the immune response and so on.

An adult builds tissue and changes his body roughly every seven years. This is of course an over-simplification, in that the brain cells cannot be replaced and bone collagen takes more like 30 years to replace, but at the other end of the scale we get a new skin every three to four weeks and two new gut linings every week. Every second, normal bone marrow makes about two and a half million new red blood cells. Every second, we create around 200,000 new immune cells, and thousands of antibody molecules. Our spares and repairs department need an awful lot of amino acid building blocks.

The amino acids
There are eight essential amino acids which are vital to life. Our friendly gut bugs make very small amounts for us all of the time, and without this background level we would suffer from severe mood swings. Antibiotics often cause mood problems as a result of loss of gut bug production.

The essential amino acids mostly lacking in plants are methionine, tryptophan and lysine. The first, methionine, is essential for a pregnant woman because a baby's thymus and immune function is dependent on it. Soya beans and legumes are deficient in methionine. All cereals are deficient in lysine.

All living things require certain amino acids more than others. Babies and children need histidine and arginine in addition to the eight essentials, and preterm babies require cysteine and taurine.

Cancer cells have their favourite diet; melanomas, for example, can be starved by withholding their chosen addiction, phenylalanine and tyrosine. The central nervous system is regulated to a large degree by amino acids, and amino acid therapy is being used increasingly in the treatment of many psychiatric disorders. In their role as neurotransmitters, proteins take on the job of vital communicators.

Amino acids are also the 'written codes' on substances, allowing the body's immune system to recognise them as self or to destroy them as rubbish or potential enemies. Antibodies, too, are protein, and lymphocytes have a high requirement for amino acids for their production and function. The amino acids which stimulate the immune system most are alanine, aspartic acid, cysteine, glycine, lysine, methionine and threonine. Those used for detoxification include glycine, methionine, cysteine, glutamine, taurine and tyrosine.

AMINO ACID THERAPY

- Alanine, carnitine, leucine, isoleucine and valine are commonly used for muscle building.
- Methionine, taurine, carnitine, arginine and glycine are used to bring down cholesterol and triglyceride levels.
- Phenylalanine, tryptophan, arginine, carnitine and gamma-amino-butyric acid (GABA) are used as appetite suppressants.
- GABA, taurine and tryptophan can be used to reduce blood pressure.
- Methionine, tryptophan and d-phenylalanine are used to control pain.
- Tryptophan, GABA and glycine relieve insomnia.
- Even serious diseases like Parkinson's disease can be helped by such amino acids as tryptophan, tyrosine, L-dopa, methionine, GABA and threonine.
- Stamina can be increased using carnitine and dimethyl glycine.

Patients with liver disease, gallbladder problems, diabetes, hypoglycaemia, aggressive behaviour, or addictions may all be helped using various combinations of amino acids. It should be remembered, however, that this is using amino acids as drugs and they should be taken under medical direction. I am a firm believer in real food. If it is eaten whole, already packaged with the nutrients it needs for its utilisation, many of these imbalances would not occur in the first place. It is very easy to create an imbalance in the body's amino acid pool, but not so easy to sort it out. For this reason I include here only a few of the amino acids, in general terms, as they apply to the immune system.

Methionine

Scientists tried to imitate what they thought was earth's primitive atmosphere. The atmosphere contained carbon, hydrogen, nitrogen, oxygen and sulphur in combination, and a spark in it formed methionine. This, plus the fact that methionine is the essential methyl donor to bacteria, leads one to conclude that it is our oldest amino acid, essential and very useful. Sunflower seeds and cottage cheese are probably the richest natural sources, and egg is also good, but potatoes are deficient.

Methionine relieves pain and is a component of various endorphins (these are chemicals involved in feelings of happiness and well being). It is very important in metabolism and enzyme systems, and essential for the foetal immune system. It is also very important for the immune systems of children; I note this, as some children are put on soya bean diets (no milk or meat), and soya bean is very deficient in methionine – in fact, it is probably the limiting factor in many soya-based infant formulae. Methionine deficiency might not be noticed until the baby grows into a more sickly child.

Experiments on monkeys show that a deficiency of methionine causes atherosclerosis. Children and pregnant mothers in particular need foods sufficient in methionine.

Cysteine and glutathione

Cysteine is very important for the immune system, mainly because it is synthesised into glutathione in the body. Its level is quite high in a normal thymus.

Millions of years before life on earth, our atmosphere was probably toxic. When life did begin, it had to develop a protection against these toxic gases. Glutathione is thought to be that protection. It is essential to our immune systems today, because, yet again, we have a lot of toxic substances in the air, both gases and heavy metals. Provided there is sufficient cysteine present, the body increases its levels of glutathione when it is trying to cope with excess lead, mercury, cadmium or arsenic; it is also thought to help with detoxification of exhaust fumes and pesticides within the body.

Glutathione is an anti-oxidant and helps protect us (and plants) against toxic forms of oxygen. It is, in fact, such a primitive and universal anti-oxidant that it has even been considered as an additive to dying lakes to restore life there. It is poorly absorbed, because there used to be sufficient of it, but a calorie-sufficient, though nutrient-deficient, modern diet may not be providing enough.

- Glutathione is necessary for macrophages, in order to make the chemicals they need to kill invaders, for lymphocyte production and for red blood cell membranes.
- Apparently, women on the pill try to produce extra glutathione, probably to protect themselves against the dangers of peroxidation of fat, as oral contraceptives are known to increase blood lipids and lipoperoxides.
- It is used in an enzyme system which lengthens fatty acid chains.
- It is synergistic with vitamins C and B_6.

With today's heavily poisoned environment, we therefore need to ensure plenty of cysteine. Reliable data on the cysteine contents of food is not readily available and vegetable sources will, in any case, vary depending on the sulphur level of the soil in which they are grown. Unfortunately, in areas which were glaciated, soil is known to be deficient in sulphur, selenium, iodine and zinc. Red peppers and eggs are the richest reliable sources of cysteine.

Threonine

Threonine is a little-known essential amino acid. It stimulates the immune system by increasing the weight and activity of the thymus and by increasing antibody production. Our treated food provides us with less threonine than we would get from natural food; for example, wild game birds provide 4 grams per pound, battery chickens only 1 g/lb; white flour does not provide any threonine, wheatgerm provides 1.35 g/lb.

Getting a balance

Correct amino acid balance is necessary for many things in the body – for good posture, strong muscles, reproduction, growth, body repair, healthy hair, healthy nails, and so on. But for the immune system, proteins, and hence amino acids, in their right balance are essential:

- To pass on a healthy and efficient immune system to your offspring.
- To make immune cells and weapons, like antibodies, with which to fight.
- To control energy levels. The correct amino acid balance is

needed at every stage of digestion, absorption and energy release. We want smooth energy levels all the time, not the high energy peaks followed by low energy troughs which result from too much sugar or refined carbohydrates and too little protein; the latter condition resembles a learner driver in first gear who has not yet worked out how to balance the clutch with the accelerator, and frog-hops down the road.

- To suppress appetite. A few amino acids directly suppress appetite when they are sufficient; if, however, they are lacking, you have a constant desire to eat.
- To control our moods. Neurotransmitters are body chemicals that make us hungry, thirsty, sexy, aggressive, angry, energetic, depressed, unhappy, etc. They control our moods and emotions, as well as our ability to learn, remember and think. Getting the amino acids right will not make anyone into a genius, but it will allow everyone to reach their full potential.
- Brain chemistry is more dependent on diet than you might think, and can be shown to alter, depending on what is eaten at the last meal: tyrosine is vital in regulating emotional moods; phenylalanine is necessary for adrenaline production and stored fat metabolism; tryptophan increases serotonin in the brain and so may relieve sleeplessness and depression; glutamine improves concentration.
- Unbalanced protein intake can increase the production of uric acid, which can lead to gout.

Many people find that when their amino acid balance is restored, they do not crave junk foods. In contrast, it is perfectly possible to live healthily and well on a vegetarian or vegan diet, although people who do so should make sure that they know how to combine amino acids; it is necessary for a range of incomplete proteins to be eaten at the same meal in order to make complete proteins in the body. In my opinion, it is not possible to live healthily and well on an entirely junk food diet, and people on this sort of diet should not only think seriously about the protein content of their food but about most of the other nutrients as well. Is a passing fancy now worth risking your future health?

CARBOHYDRATES

Carbohydrates make up the greater part of our diet and are obtained from grains, fruit, vegetables, legumes, nuts and most processed foods.

Complex carbohydrates are much the best way to obtain these, as they come complete with the nutrients necessary for their utilisation. They are a bit like time-release capsules. Simple sugars and refined carbohydrates flood the system with sugars as soon as they are absorbed; this provides a quick flash of energy, but it is followed by a long period of lethargy. In contrast, complex carbohydrates release their sugars slowly so that the level of sugar in the blood remains roughly within a normal range, instead of going up and down like a seesaw. An average blood sugar level is around 90 milligrams/100 ml of blood. If this is maintained, energy levels are good. When it gets down to 70 mg/100 ml the biochemistry alters to tell us that we are hungry – amino acid communication. At 65 mg/100 ml we crave sweets and become easily irritated, moody and uncooperative. If sufficient and appropriate food is eaten, we feel fine, think quickly and clearly, lose our hunger pangs, and even find sweets distasteful.

Starch
Starch is the fundamental carbohydrate we consume, and can be obtained from grains, bread, pulses and vegetables like potato.

We should try to be a little more adventurous with our grains. Although we appear to have a wide variety of foods, our national addiction is definitely wheat. Pastas, pizzas, pastries, biscuits, pies, bread and cakes are all apparently different foods when seen on the menu, but in reality are all wheat. Even breakfast cereals 'specialise' in wheat.

Because of this, our immune system views our 'varied' diet as monotonous. It likes a change, so that it does not get fed up with wheat and does not start attacking it. Try barley, rye, rice, corn (maize) and millet sometimes. Choose wholegrain breakfast cereals rather than sugar- and salt-laden refined ones, and eat lots of vegetables, both raw and cooked.

It is a good habit to eat a few raw vegetables as a starter before a cooked meal. This helps your immune system to deal with the following food without having such a fight. It used to be thought that digestive leucocytosis, i.e. migration of white blood cells to the gut wall and their subsequent destruction, occurred whenever and what-ever we ate, but it has now been found that this migration of white blood cells to the gut and their destruction only occurs when we eat cooked food. Raw food does not waste immune soldiers, and raw food before a cooked meal lessens the overall destruction of white blood cells.

Just as starch is the carbohydrate storage compound in plants, so glycogen is the carbohydrate storage compound in animals (including humans). But we get very little glycogen in our diet as it is broken down to glucose after the death of an animal. Meat therefore contains sugar. It is especially important for those involved in a lot of physical activity to eat complex carbohydrate, which is then stored as glycogen and can be used for physical energy when required.

Sugars

We need sugars, glucose is the final breakdown product of all carbohydrate and it is what we, and especially our brains, need as a food. But sugars have got a bad name, mainly because our intake is again out of balance with our needs. At present, one-third of our intake of carbohydrate in the United Kingdom is in the form of sucrose – the sugar we buy in the shops. This 'food' provides nothing except energy, and gets stored as saturated fat if it is not used. Much of it is hidden in highly processed foods and drinks, invisible but actively destructive. As we eat nearly 60 per cent of our calories as carbohydrates, we must be eating nearly 20 per cent of our total calorie intake in the form of sucrose. At least, some people are. In fact, some must be eating more than a fifth of their diet as sucrose, to make up for those of us who avoid it as much as possible.

Sucrose is not only nutrient free: it actually requires nutrients for its metabolism, so it has to steal them from somewhere else. It is one of the reasons why vitamin B deficiency is so common. We waste precious nutrients including the B vitamins trying to process this useless sugar. Although sugar is less alien to the immune system than artificial sweeteners, the problem is that we are eating too much of it. Small amounts are fine; but one-fifth of our daily diet is excessive.

Carbohydrates make up the bulk of plant material, and constitute anything from 40 per cent (affluent people) to 90 per cent (poor and protein-deficient people) of our diet. The optimum intake is probably somewhere around 50-60 per cent, preferably consumed in its natural form, complete with fibre and nutrients.

FIBRE

Fibre is calorie free and good for slimming as it passes through the system without being digested; it fills you up without giving you anything with which to form fat. But a high-fibre diet does not mean sprinkling bran on everything; in fact, this habit can cause more problems than it solves. If bran is your way to get fibre, then take all your bran at one meal only, and take your nutrient-packed foods at other meals. Remember that wheat bran is a refined food, just like white flour; whole foods are a better way to take fibre. Many people sensitive to wheat bran could try oat and rice bran.

Dry cereal like cereal fibre goes in at one end and comes out at the other, and does a scouring job in between. If it is taken regularly, preferably as a whole grain, it reduces the build-up of faecal material, and so helps the absorption of nutrients through the intestine. A lifetime on a low-fibre diet will create a much thicker faecal build-up in the intestines, and so absorption of nutrients will be less. Minerals, however, do tend to be attracted to fibre, so eating fibre with every meal can actually leave you mineral deficient. This is another good example of the need to get the balance right.

There are many types of fibre. Gums, resins and pectins, as well as cellulose, which is the major component of plant cell walls, all provide fibre. Ruminant animals can break cellulose down into sugars, but we cannot do this. However, the bugs in our gut do need it in order to stay healthy. So eating greens keeps our welcome guests happy and, in return, they keep us clean and tidy inside and provide us with a bonus of B vitamins, essential amino acids and fats. What a bargain.

A clean gut is obviously better for the immune system. If we are repeatedly constipated, there is a build-up of toxins which can be absorbed into the bloodstream; the immune system has to deal with this. And no self-respecting bugs want to live in a constipated gut. They move out and make room for the less reputable varieties, like candida, who are willing to slum it in these unhealthy living conditions.

Faulty fibre intake does not become obvious immediately; it may be 20 or 40 years later that the problems are revealed.

16
VITAMINS AND MINERALS

It was only at the end of the last century that people realised that there was more to food than just carbohydrate, fat and protein, although Egyptian doctors had earlier prescribed liver as a cure for night blindness. It is now known that deficiency or excess of many of the vitamins and minerals cause the body to malfunction.

The obvious single deficiency diseases like scurvy, beri-beri and pellagra are rare nowadays. We suffer more from marginal deficiencies of several vitamins. This makes life more complicated, because specific deficiency symptoms are not obvious; they overlap and so are difficult to diagnose.

Vitamin excesses are much less common; the causes include taking too many supplements, taking them out of balance with one another, or having a narrow diet which contains too much of one or two specific foods. It is quite rare to find a single food which contains an excess of any one micronutrient. Polar bear liver is one example; it contains such a high level of vitamin A that it would be toxic to eat a normal portion. It is, however, possible to go on silly diets that require you to eat all one food, which could mimic this sort of condition. A good nutritional balance cannot be achieved using these diets.

This chapter considers the vitamins and minerals we need, what they do for your immune system, deficiency symptoms, supplementation and usual food sources. However, it must he remembered that the nutrient content of food depends on the soil in which it has been grown, and the method of storing, spraying and other general forms of human interference. Having to take supplements to make up for what should be in food is often necessary but makes the food not only expensive but difficult to balance. The sooner the food industry gets back to real food, the better. Unfortunately, this is unlikely, as profit comes before health (the increased national health bill caused by deficient food comes out of a different purse).

There is no one dosage of food supplements for everyone; we all have different requirements. The following is intended for information, not prescription. Individual supplementation depends on diet, lifestyle, health, medication and a whole host of other circumstances which would need to be taken into consideration when advising any individual. If, however, anyone feels the need to supplement their diet with vitamins and minerals in excess of the recommended dosage, it is best to seek professional advice, as you can quite easily unbalance your system. More is not always better.

REASONS FOR NUTRIENT DEFICIENCIES

- We tend to eat more processed food, rather than whole foods, and many necessary nutrients are lost in the processing. This may include some essential nutrients that have yet to be discovered.
- Refined foods still need vitamins for their utilisation in the body; if these are not provided with the food, they have to be taken from body stores or the food is not utilised properly.
- Soil depletion over the years has led to deficient crops.
- Toxic sprays used on crops can further deplete our body stores.
- Increased shelf life or storage reduces vitamin content.
- Food is often harvested before it has reached its peak vitamin content.
- Artificial chemicals and additives to food deplete the vitamin content of both the food and the body stores.
- Home cooking or preserving causes vitamin loss.
- The state of health of the person may affect their vitamin utilisation; for example, a diabetic cannot convert beta-carotene to vitamin A, so they need their supply of vitamin A preformed, that is, as cod liver oil rather than as carrots. Similarly, people with gut problems like diverticular disease, irritable bowel syndrome, etc., cannot absorb vitamins as efficiently as those with healthy guts.
- It has also been established that the ability to absorb vitamins and minerals is reduced as we age.
- Drugs can increase the requirements for some vitamins and destroy others.

VITAMIN A

This is known as the growth vitamin, because it is necessary for the production of the growth hormone, which in turn is responsible, not only for growth, but for maintaining an active thymus and hence a strong immune system. T cells will obviously be depleted if growth hormone is in short supply as the thymus will have shrunk, it will be less active and so will be less efficient at maturing T cells. B cells are also adversely affected.

Vitamin A is a powerful antiviral vitamin, mainly because its inclusion in cell walls makes them stronger and more resistant to viral attack. It is particularly important for strong linings in areas of special risk from infection, such as the respiratory system, the gut and the genito-urinary tract.

Body secretions like sweat, tears and saliva, as well as the immune system's cells, all contain lysozyme and need vitamin A for the production of this protective antibacterial enzyme. Along with vitamin C, vitamin A is probably deficient in individuals who regularly suffer from conjunctivitis.

Vitamin A's precursor, beta-carotene, is being researched because of its possible role in preventing and treating cancer and for use after major surgery.

Vitamin A and beta-carotene must combine with bile salts in the gut in order to pass into the bloodstream. If someone is on a very low fat diet, bile does not reach the intestine and over 90 per cent of the vitamin A may be lost in the faeces. Furthermore, vitamin E intake is crucial, to prevent destruction of vitamin A before it can be utilised or stored.

Foods usually rich in vitamin A or its precursor beta-carotene

Foods containing beta-carotene
- All green vegetables, such as spinach, cabbage, endive, lettuce, kale, broccoli, legumes (cashew nuts and beans).
- Carrots, swedes, corn, pumpkin, sweet potato and peppers.
- Cherries, canteloupe melon, water melon, peach and papayas.

Foods containing vitamin A
- Eggs.
- Milk fat, butter, cream.
- Fish oils and oily fish.
- Liver, kidney.

When we may need more of these
- If suffering from an infection, especially a viral infection.
- If suffering from cystic fibrosis.
- If suffering from atherosclerosis.
- If diabetic, you would need preformed vitamin A. More care is needed not to over-supplement the preformed variety.
- If the system is coping with an intake of mineral oil, perhaps as a laxative. (It is not a good idea to consume mineral oil, see Chapter 14.)
- If deficient in protein, as vitamin A is needed for its synthesis.
- If the diet is rich in protein, as protein requires vitamin A for its utilisation.
- If vegetables, fruit and fish are not a major part of the diet.
- If suffering from skin conditions (psoriasis, acne, etc.)
- If you smoke; the mucous lining of the respiratory tract is damaged by smoke and lots of vitamin A is used up in repairs.
- If you live in a heavily polluted area – exhaust fumes destroy vitamin A.
- If bladder stones are a problem.
- If you are under a lot of stress, which will increase adrenal activity and decrease the thymus. Vitamin A is needed to reverse this.
- During winter the body is less able to utilise vitamin A in cold conditions. Perhaps this is why the polar bear stores so much. It is protective against hypothermia for elderly people; it is important that they take extra during the winter months.
- Males who are impotent may suffer from vitamin A deficiency.
- Alcoholics need extra vitamin A.
- If you have been exposed to a carcinogen, the waiting period (preneoplasia), which may be up to 20 years from exposure to the manifestation of cancer, is probably the time when vitamin A exerts most of its protective effect and prevents malignancy.

Possible symptoms of deficiency
- Poor growth in children.
- Poor night vision.
- Mouth ulcers.
- Skin complaints, from dandruff to acne.
- Genito-urinary infections or vaginitis, especially in the elderly.
- Susceptibility to viral infections in general.
- Decline in sense of taste, smell and hearing.
- Lack of tears and extreme sensitivity to light.
- Improper tooth and bone formation.

Supplements

When supplements of vitamin A are needed, they are best taken in the form of beta-carotene as this form is not toxic and is only made into vitamin A as required. Diabetics need preformed vitamin A or cod liver oil as they cannot convert beta-carotene into vitamin A. If children do not like vitamin A-containing foods, they may prefer cod liver oil, but they only need this during the winter.

Dosage varies from person to person, depending on the diet, life-style and condition. Up to 20,000 international units (iu) beta-carotene can be regularly used. This is usually lowered to 10,000 iu when pregnant. Supplements need to be taken with a little fat and vitamin E to be effective.

B COMPLEX VITAMINS

B vitamins are essential for bacteria, so do not bother to take supplements during a bacterial infection. They are also important most of the time for every cell of the body, and that includes those of the immune system, where they build better resistance. They are particularly important for mucous membranes. Folic acid and pyridoxine (B_6) probably have the most effect on the immune function.

Folic acid is essential for pregnant mothers and for the development of mature organs of the foetus. It has been found that the thymus is larger and the immune system stronger if the mother has had a good supply of folic acid, choline, B_{12} and methionine. Folic acid is also necessary for all cell division, and hence is of particular importance, not only for the infant, but also whenever there is a need for healing.

A B_6 deficiency causes a decrease in the activity of the phagocytic cells so that we cannot clean up inside as effectively as we should.

Choline is another important B vitamin, in that it changes into dimethyl-glycine in the body. This substance increases lymphocyte production three or four times in comparison with a deficient animal. It is also a natural detoxification supplement.

Food sources

Major food sources are liver, yeast, blackstrap molasses, whole grains and, especially, wheatgerm and rice bran.

- B_1: Offal, pork, beef, whole grains, nuts, legumes and sunflower seeds.
- B_2: Liver, milk, meat, leafy green vegetables and sunflower seeds.

- B_3: Organ meats, meat, peanuts, legumes, milk, eggs, tuna and sunflower seeds.
- Folic acid: Dark green vegetables, organ meat, beans, whole grains, salmon, tuna, dates and milk.
- B_6: Molasses, offal, whole grains, green vegetables, peas and prunes.
- B_{12}: Milk and dairy produce, fish, offal and eggs.
- B_5: Yeast, green vegetables (especially broccoli), cashew nuts, milk, eggs, mushrooms, nuts, salmon and seeds.
- Para-amino benzoic acid (PABA): Offal, eggs, whole grains and yeast.
- Choline: fish, eggs, offal, yeast and peanuts.
- Biotin: Organ meats, molasses and milk.
- Inositol: Organ meats, molasses, whole grains, nuts.
- Pantothenic acid: Yeast, whole grains, meat, organ meats, nuts, peas, beans, dates and cauliflower.

When we need more B vitamins
- Women suffering from premenstrual tension (PMT) often need more.
- Pregnancy or the use of oral contraceptives increases the need for folic acid and B_6.
- Conclusion of a course of antibiotics.
- Pantothenic acid (B_5) is often deficient in allergic bottle-fed babies.
- Hypoglycaemics need extra pantothenic acid.
- Heavy refined-sugar eaters need more B complex; in fact heavy eaters in general need a lot of B vitamins, especially if consuming refined foods.
- Anyone taking cortisone is probably deficient in B_5.
- Really overweight people who fast or who drastically cut down on food without adding B vitamins, especially B_5, can get symptoms of arthritis or gout.
- Alcoholics are B deficient.
- The adrenal glands can produce sex hormones; these are invaluable to a woman after the menopause, and help to prevent osteoporosis, as long as they are not exhausted by excess tea and coffee drinking combined with a deficiency of pantothenic acid.
- Tannin in tea is an anti-B_1 agent; heavy tea drinkers need more B vitamins.
- Radiotherapy sickness is sometimes alleviated using B_6 with a low dose B complex under medical supervision.

- Children on soya-milk diets are often B deficient, B_2 in particular. It first manifests itself as red, watery eyes.
- People with high cholesterol levels require extra niacin.
- Those who suffer with indigestion daily are often B deficient and cannot make the hydrochloric acid necessary for digestion in the stomach.

Possible symptoms of deficiency
The B vitamins are used by just about every cell in the body, and they are used in a lot of the body's chemistry, so their deficiency symptoms are very varied, although almost always there are mental effects such as depression, anxiety, difficulty with concentration and moodiness. There is often also an energy problem, because B vitamins are needed to make energy from food; without them, lack of energy or tiredness are inevitable.

A host of other symptoms may also be evident, like headaches, pre menstrual tension (PMT), bad breath, dandruff, eczema, water retention, weight problems, sensitivity to light and so on.

Probably one of the most reliable physical guides to B vitamin inadequacies is the mouth, and in particular the tongue: cracked sore lips and mouth corners; tongue enlargement or decrease in the size of the tongue itself or of the taste buds on it; deep fissures or, alternatively, a very smooth sore tongue; coatings, smell or off-colour tongues are all telling you that you are B deficient. The obvious deficiency in the mouth will be extended to other areas of digestion. Stomach acid production and enzymes will be insufficient and the chances are there will be excessive gas and indigestion.

Gut bugs also need B vitamins to do their housework in the intestines; without their contribution, this area will not be as well kept as it could be and, after a long period of deficiency, could well become a slum area.

Supplements
If it is necessary to supplement the diet, it is better to take a B complex, including a good balance of them all. Taking one or two only increases the need for the others, and having a poor balance can create as many problems as it may solve; vitamin B_2 and B_6 intake in particular must be about even.

A B50 complex is a usual supplement, containing 50 mg of each of the main B family. B100s may be necessary for a period if there is severe deficiency or if a course of antibiotics have just been finished

– medication such as antibiotics, sulphonamides and others destroy
B vitamins.

Sometimes a single B vitamin is supplemented for a short time to
restore a balance. It should always be taken with a low dose B
complex or with plenty of B-rich food.

WHAT DOES VITAMIN C DO FOR THE IMMUNE SYSTEM?

- Vitamin C is antiviral. Many viruses such as flu and the
  common cold do not penetrate deeply into the body and
  do not normally enter the bloodstream. They spread from
  cell to cell in the mucous secretions on the respiratory
  tract membranes. Consequently there is very little antibody stimulation. Defence falls to cell-mediated
  T lymphocytes only. The vitamin C level of T lymphocytes is depleted by smoking, age and infection; supplementation in these cases increases the ability of T
  lymphocytes to do their job and, in the latter case, reduces
  the symptoms.
- Prostaglandin E production in blood platelets is boosted
  by vitamin C, and this in turn increases the T-lymphocyte
  production. The greater the number and effectiveness of
  an army, the better the chance of victory.
- Vitamin C is needed for a special kind of cell division
  called phytohaemagglutinin-induced blastogenesis, which
  results in a rapid increase in lymphocytes of both B-cell
  and T-cell types. The flu virus actually works by
  depressing this cell division. Vitamin C supplementation
  switches it back on again. However, the dose needed to do
  this is 3 to 5 grams a day, depending on the individual.
- Interferon production is greater with sufficient vitamin C.
  It is produced by the infected cell and causes a further
  protein to be produced by itself and neighbouring cells
  which blocks the synthesis of essential viral proteins. As
  viruses cannot replicate themselves, but need the host cell
  to do it for them, it stands to reason that the greater the
  production of interferon, the less cells will make the virus.
- Vitamin C can be bacteriostatic or bactericidal, depending
  on the bug. Most bacteria require B vitamins for their life
  processes, but not vitamin C – the latter can seriously

hinder bacterial growth and multiplication. It can even kill some bacteria under the right conditions.

- C_3 complement production is improved with vitamin C and this in turn triggers B lymphocytes to manufacture more antibodies, especially IgA, IgG and IgM.
- It stimulates non-lysozyme antibacterial factor (NLAF) found in tears. This is of obvious importance for people who often suffer from eye infections.
- Vitamin C enables those leucocytes responsible for engulfing foreign particles to carry out their function. Leucocytes can only perform phagacytosis if they contain at least 20 micrograms of vitamin C per 100 million cells.
- Vitamin C detoxifies, partially at least, many bacterial toxins, depending on the bug involved. It is often the toxin which causes all the unpleasant symptoms.
- Apart from stimulating natural antibacterial factors in the body, vitamin C will actually improve the performance of antibiotics.
- Mononuclear phagocytes, a special type of leucocyte or white blood cell, use vitamin C with hydrogen peroxide and some minerals, especially zinc, to kill the invaders that they have captured. Research shows that zinc has a role to play in the prevention of colds, especially if sucked slowly with vitamin C.
- Vitamin C also helps sore eyes and runny nose, as it is a natural antihistamine.
- Vitamin C obviously has a great effect on the immune system, but dose is important – it will vary from individual to individual. If a cold or any other form of infection catches you, increase your supply until it is over, then gradually decrease your dosage again.

VITAMIN C

Most animals have an enzyme called L-guconolactone oxidase which allows them to make vitamin C. Man, along with guinea pigs, the Indian fruit-eating bat and the red vented bulbul bird, do not. All these rely on vitamin C in their diet and all die of scurvy without it. Man can make very small amounts from folic acid, because folic acid is converted in the body to its biologically active form, tetrahydrofolic acid and ascorbic acid; unfortunately folic acid is also commonly found to be deficient and only supplied in micro amounts, so we get very little vitamin C this way.

Irwin Stone, an eminent biochemist, postulated that during evolution man lost his ability to make this ascorbic acid in sufficient quantities due to a mutation in the gene that makes the particular liver enzyme L-guconolactone oxidase. He suggested that the mutation did not pose any threat at that time, because man was a great fruit eater and had plenty of vitamin C in the diet; now, however, it is a different matter. Storage and processing deplete our food of vitamin C, and we eat less fresh fruit than our ancestors did. Other animals, like the gorilla, living in the wild, consume about 4.5 grams of vitamin C daily in fresh food. Other mammals too, saturate blood and tissue with vitamin C and step up their production when they are ill or under stress. It is possible that infectious diseases, cardiovascular disorders, collagen diseases, cancer and premature aging are among the many ills which could be prevented if we still had the ability to regulate our vitamin C levels.

Whilst many studies confirm benefits with supplemental vitamin C, others do not, probably due to the fact that the dosage has to be sufficient for any given person at any given time – it is very difficult to judge the correct amount.

Bowel tolerance is a useful general indication of vitamin C requirements. A normal, young, healthy adult will tolerate 1 to 4 g of vitamin C before getting diarrhoea. If the patient has flu, this tolerance may go up to 4 to 8 g, while if he has cancer or AIDS, he may require 20 to 30 g a day. It all depends on the individual, which makes research a little more difficult. Age is another major factor; our absorption of vitamin C goes down considerably with age, though in old animals its production is not that much different to that in young animals. Older people need more vitamin C spread out in small amounts over the day.

Needless to say, a lot of work has been done on guinea pigs as they most closely resemble us as far as vitamin C utilisation is concerned. For example in very low vitamin C diets, cholesterol formation in their adrenal glands went up 600 per cent and their ability to heal wounds was poor.

It is known that during phagocytosis oxygen is used up, hydrogen peroxide is produced and used to destroy the germ which has been captured and the hexose monophosphate shunt (the chemical process whereby the cell gets more energy from glucose) is speeded up. Researchers have found that this activity is low in normal, healthy white blood cells, but is speeded up, by up to six times the norm, when they are infected. The speed was greater when vitamin C was added. In those with scurvy or those who are vitamin C deficient, the white blood cells engulf bacteria but cannot digest them or destroy them. Vitamin C reverses this cellular indigestion.

Food sources
Most fresh fruits are very good sources of vitamin C, especially oranges, kiwi and melon, as long as they have not been kept in storage for too long.

Most vegetables are also good sources, especially greens, tomatoes and peppers.

When you may need more
- During the winter intake may be stepped up for protection against colds and flu; and it should be stepped up a lot if exposed to these viruses or if initial symptoms are felt.
- Those who both smoke and drink alcohol need more vitamin C as it is known to help detoxify acetaldehyde. Smokers on average have 25 per cent less vitamin C in the blood than similar non-smokers who are on the same diet. Heavy drinkers also need extra vitamin C and zinc as both are necessary for the production of alcohol dehydrogenase, the liver enzyme which detoxifies alcohol.
- Diabetics cannot transport vitamin C across cell membranes very well, and side effects such as poor wound healing can be helped by supplements of vitamin C.
- Aspirin depletes the body's vitamin C reserves, so these should be replenished by those on aspirin therapy.
- The need for vitamin C in the diet increases with age.
- High cholesterol levels may be lowered with sufficient vitamin C. Research shows that a normal guinea pig converts 40 per cent more cholesterol to a safer form than does one which is deficient in vitamin C. It also tends to have less atherosclerosis than deficient ones.
- Most medical drugs destroy vitamin C in the body, although many of them are first detoxified by it. The destructive effect, however, may go on for some weeks after the drug is discontinued. Drugs are sometimes necessary and life saving, so it is probably wise to increase vitamin C intake if you have to take them.

Possible symptoms of deficiency
- Easy bruising.
- Bleeding or receding gums.
- Slow healing.
- Frequent infections.

Supplementation

Supplements are best taken with bioflavonoids, or food containing them. Vitamin C or ascorbic acid powder is the cheapest and purest form in which to buy this, as it does not have the fillers and binders which would be needed to make tablets. If ascorbic acid is not well tolerated by the stomach (it sometimes causes heartburn), the more gentle calcium ascorbate can be used; this is not acidic, and can be mixed with water, or orange juice in the same way.

Many people like to take vitamin C daily, but it can also be used as a 'medicine' by increasing the dosage if illness does threaten. Always remember to take it with a lot of fluid and to decrease the intake gradually when an infection has passed, rather than to stop suddenly.

VITAMIN D

Vitamin D, when taken in excess, suppresses the immune system. People who suffer from conditions that already suppress their immune system are generally advised to avoid supplementation. However, it must be remembered that vitamin D is essential for healthy bones, and hence for normal movement. Indirectly the immune system suffers if bones are unhealthy and you cannot move freely.

Japanese studies show that a daily supplement of around 500 iu of the natural form of vitamin D_3 may help to reverse the disturbed helper/suppressor T-cell ratio which occurs in ME (myalgic encephalomyelitis).

I am a firm believer in sunshine for many reasons, and this is one. When the sun's ultraviolet light hits the skin, it changes a form of cholesterol in the skin into cholecalciferol, which is the natural form of vitamin D (also known as D_3). Other Ds, namely D_2, D_4, D_5 and D_6, are synthetic versions and have greater side effects than the natural D_3 (which is also found in fish oil).

Our skin colour determines the amount of ultraviolet light (UV) we let through and the amount of vitamin D made. Black skin only allows 3 to 36 per cent of the UV through, whilst white skin allows 52 to 72 per cent to be absorbed. As white skin tans, the amount of UV allowed through is reduced, so offering protection from damage which could cause skin cancer, and regulating the amount of vitamin D made. In general, we make less vitamin D in winter, because we have less exposure to sunlight; supplemental fish oil during the winter months is therefore quite a good idea for children and the elderly in particular, because bone needs calcium, magnesium and vitamin D for growth and repair. Many of the degenerative bone problems could be avoided with the right diet, exercise and exposure to sunshine, but that is another story.

Suffice it to say that the immune system is healthier for movement. For pain-free movement we need strong healthy bones. We also need to have the immune system suppressed sometimes. After an infection has passed, for example, we need to be able to turn off the immune system; this requires suppressors. It is the right balance that we are aiming for, and the right amount of vitamin D is needed to play its part.

Main food sources
- Cod liver or halibut liver oils.
- Oily fish.
- Egg yolk.
- Milk.

When you may need more
- If already suffering from osteoporosis or degeneration of the spine.
- If you spend a lot of time indoors or are bedridden.

Supplements
Natural supplements like fish oil are the best.

Vitamin D is fat soluble and so is stored in the body. It is possible to take too much, so sunlight and fish should be used wherever possible and only supplemented when really necessary.

VITAMIN E

Unfortunately, these days we seem to be obsessed by increasing the shelf life of foods so that they keep longer than the people who eat them. Vitamin E is an essential nutrient, but it is often removed if the food is to be kept for a long time; although a natural antioxidant, it goes off faster than artificial ones which are used to replace it.

Vitamin E is necessary for a normal antibody response. As an anti-oxidant in our fat layers. it neutralises free radicals and works with other nutrients to improve our resistance to infection. It is very effective in protecting us from air pollution, particularly that due to exhausts, air purifiers or deodorisers which generate ozone.

Main food sources
- Whole grains – rice, wheat, wheatgerm, oats.
- Cold-pressed oils – sunflower, safflower.
- Green leafy vegetables.
- Eggs and liver.

Supplements
Supplements should be built up gradually, 100 iu at a time, to a maximum of 1,000 iu. Although good for heart complaints, people suffering from these should be especially wary to include this vitamin only gradually and with professional advice. Vitamin E may reduce the need for drugs like anticoagulants.

MINERALS

As you might expect, essential minerals are all necessary for immune function and enzyme systems, while the toxic ones inhibit the immune system.

Mineral in this book is used to include any element, metal or non-metal, because it is a popular term which most people understand. This is not chemically correct however, as minerals are really compounds; salt, for example, is a mineral, a compound of sodium and chlorine – sodium chloride.

My intention is to cover only those minerals of special importance to the immune system.

CALCIUM

Calcium is very important for the immune system. All phagocytic cells need calcium, and they absorb more of it whenever antigens are present. They use it to make the enzymes which are necessary to destroy the invader once they have engulfed it. Calcium is also used for attachment and ingestion of an invader by the macrophages.

Without calcium we cannot use one of our major defences against invasion – the classical pathway for complement fixation (Chapters 4 and 5).

Calcium is needed for fever production. Fever offers us many advantages when our immune defences are at war. Macrophages move faster and produce enzymes faster when they are at a temperature slightly above normal body temperature. It is also significant that some viruses cannot replicate at this elevated temperature and others cannot function at all. Fever puts them at a disadvantage and us at an advantage, as long as, of course, the temperature does not go too high.

Cytotoxic T cells require calcium to make their killing enzymes.

Food sources
- Milk, cheese and dairy produce.
- Beans, soya beans, peanuts and seeds.
- Fish, especially those with bones which you can eat.
- Grains and bread.

Absorption is prevented by:
- High-fat diets.
- Too much phytic acid found in grains.
- Too much oxalic acid found in rhubarb and chocolate.
- Insufficient vitamin D or sunshine.
- Presence of too many toxic minerals such as aluminium and lead.
- Various gut conditions – diverticular disease, etc.

High-protein diets increase the loss of calcium.

MAGNESIUM

This is a much needed, yet frequently forgotten, mineral. It is often deficient these days, causing many health problems including heart conditions.

It is needed for the alternative pathway for complement fixation. With negligible calcium and magnesium intake, complement fixation – a whole defence system in its own right – can be entirely lost.

Magnesium is also needed for cell-mediated immunity, maintaining thymus and antibody levels.

A magnesium deficiency may cause a rise in histamine, and hence in allergic reactions.

It is important that calcium, magnesium and phosphorus are kept in balance. Unfortunately, fast food and soft drink diets are very high in phosphorus. Furthermore, the increasing awareness of the problem of osteoporosis has meant that many people now take extra calcium whilst magnesium is neglected. This lack of magnesium, but increased calcium and phosphorus, can cause an increase in arthritic pain and calcification in tissues where calcification is not desirable.

Food sources
- Nuts.
- Green vegetables.
- Corn.
- Some fruit, e.g. apples, figs and citrus fruits.
- Seeds – sesame seed has one of the best balances of calcium and magnesium. It is necessary to grind them to ensure the breaking of the seed to release the minerals.
- Water in hard-water areas. Note: water softeners and filters remove calcium and magnesium from the water.

Supplements
The supplement range is 200 to 500 mg.

If you increase calcium, you should also increase magnesium. Milk of Magnesia or Epsom salts may be used in very small amounts (not at laxative levels), but should not be taken with a protein meal as it neutralises the acid needed for digestion. Dolomite is also a source if you can get it free of lead and cadmium.

IRON

Iron is essential for antibody production. It is required by red blood cells and to make the killing enzymes used by PMSs and macrophages. The intracellular enzyme, myeloperoxidase, contains iron and is used in the formation of white blood cells.

Bacteria, however, usually cannot reproduce without iron, so when suffering from a bacterial infection, discontinue any iron supplement. The leucocytes produce an iron-binding protein when there is a bacterial infection, and there is no sense in overworking it.

Iron deficiency is common in children, menstruating women and some vegetarians, but it is not a good idea to over-supplement as too much can suppress the immune system. We are back again to the magic balance; unfortunately, our food is so altered these days that it is difficult to know if you are getting enough. Many people dislike offal and greens, which are rich sources.

Main food sources
- Meat, especially offal.
- Green vegetables.
- Cereals.
- Bread.
- Egg yolk.
- Peaches.

SELENIUM

British soil levels are low in selenium, and our cancer levels are quite high. There may well be a link. It is known that selenium levels are often low in cancer patients, and selenium is believed to offer protection from cancer-causing substances. It is a very good anti-oxidant, working with vitamin E. It is used in antibody production, and white blood cells seem to lose their ability to recognise invaders without it.

However, we only need around 50 micrograms (μg) per day, and more is definitely not better – too much can be toxic. Natural food sources are nuts, cereals, seafoods, and vegetables or fruit grown in selenium-rich soil.

ZINC

Zinc is not really stored in the body, but deficiency causes atrophy of the thymus, possibly due to the fact that it prevents normal release of vitamin A from the liver. (Vitamin A and zinc work together.)

It is needed for enzymes which destroy cancer cells. However, too much is not advised when cancer is established or when there is a viral infection as zinc is needed for cells to replicate. The right amount of zinc is beneficial for cancer sufferers, especially for odour problems in terminal cases.

White spots in the nails, a decline in the sense of smell or taste, and poor wound healing are indications of a poor zinc status and is quite common where water pipes are made of copper. It is important that zinc and copper are in the right balance; an excess or deficiency of one or the other can cause immune and other problems.

Zinc is found in over 200 of the body's enzymes. The hormone thymulin, which is necessary for maturation of T-cells, is one of those dependent on zinc.

Zinc is lost with seminal fluid, so men with high sexual activity could become deficient. Adolescents, with their change in hormone production, also need more than usual, as do pregnant women, especially if carrying a male child.

Supplementation should be at a level of 15 mg a day when there is a deficiency.

Food sources
- Meat, organ meats.
- Shellfish.
- Eggs.
- Leafy green vegetables.
- Seeds, especially pumpkin seeds.

CONCLUSION

Vitamins and minerals all work together with the food we eat to make strong, healthy, optimally functioning bodies. Sometimes it may be necessary to take one specific nutrient for a period of time to correct a deficiency, but it should not normally be necessary to take large doses of a single vitamin or mineral for long periods, as it could put the rest out of balance.

Nutrient-deficient food is common nowadays, as is food laden with undesirable chemicals. This increases the need for balanced food supplements, although these should not be taken as substitutes for real food. If you can find whole food that has nothing added and nothing taken away, eat it: but also be aware of what your body needs. Our nutrient needs alter many times during our lives. Sometimes we need more of one nutrient, sometimes more of another. Symptoms and circumstances will indicate which. Nutrient-packed foods are essential for good health, devitalised ones are unnecessary; supplements are useful for correcting inbalances and enabling us to reach our optimum health and vitality.

17
PREPARING AND COOKING FOR HEALTH

This chapter is all about getting the most nutrients out of real everyday food and guiding reluctant immune boosters into a healthier path. It is a collection of useful facts about whole foods. It is not meant as a complete guide to healthy eating, just as a taster of the richer, more lasting treasures in store when you turn to foods in natural, rather than cardboard, tin, aluminium, glass or plastic, containers. We are very fortunate in this country to have ample good food. We should use it wisely rather than strip it of its valuable nutrients.

VEGETABLES

Everyone knows that vegetables are healthy. They contain varying amounts of protein and carbohydrates, but little, if any, fat; any fat present is usually unsaturated. Fresh vegetables are high in vitamins and minerals, although a variety is needed to cover the whole range. Their water content is high and their calorific value is usually low. They contain plenty of fibre.

Choosing vegetables

Generally most vegetables should be firm, not soft. A leafy vegetable should not be limp, but able to hold itself up. Colour is important in revealing freshness; usually the darker the intended colour, the higher the vitamin content (although sometimes coloured lights are used in shops to disguise poor colour). Washed vegetables may have lost some of their nutritional value, depending on how long they have been left in the water and whether the water contained any chemicals. Buy dirty ones from choice and wash them at home just before use.

Vegetables which have been grown next to a busy road, or are displayed in a shop near a busy road, may well contain a lead supplement from the car exhaust fumes. Much of this can be removed by washing in a weak vinegar solution and then rinsing with fresh water. Organically grown vegetables are obviously preferable if you can find and afford them.

Vegetables lose vitamins, not minerals, on storage, as do most foods. All vegetables store better in the cool and dark. Some vitamins, in particular B_2 and B_6, are destroyed by light. Root vegetables, bought by the sack, need dry conditions. Leafy vegetables are probably best in the fridge. Food bought in season has the best nutrient content; forced vegetables have inferior nutritional qualities and are often much higher in nitrates. Nitrites and nitrates destroy beta-carotene, our vegetable form of vitamin A, both in the growing food and in the body; they prevent it from ever forming vitamin A.

Preparing vegetables
- Cook in skins if possible, even if you then peel them before eating. The skin will keep minerals in during cooking and, in any case, can be peeled much more thinly after cooking. Skins provide vital fibre, but unfortunately, they also contain residues of any chemical spray. Compromise – eat the fibre and pesticides one day and peel them off the next.
- Do not leave vegetables soaking in water. This leaches out the B and C vitamins, in particular, and also allows more fat to be taken up if the vegetables are to be fried afterwards, as in the case of chips, for example.
- When boiling, put the vegetables straight into boiling, not cold, water. If they are put into cold water and heated to boiling, there will be more enzyme destruction, as well as more colour and vitamin loss. Use the minimum amount of water. Vegetables do not need to be covered by the water, as long as a lid is used to hold in the steam.
- Add any salt right at the end of cooking and do not use sodium bicarbonate at all. Both of these increase the loss of nutrients, especially vitamin C, as well as colour and flavour.
- Do not use aluminium pans as acidic ingredients will dissolve the aluminium and this will go into the food. Copper utensils will also accelerate oxidation and increase the loss of vitamin C. Stainless steel or glass utensils seem to do the least harm.
- Stainless steel pressure cookers are very good for retaining nutrients, with the exception of vitamin B_1; this vitamin is stable with dry heat, but not moist heat, so foods rich in B_1 are better

cooked in an oven without water.

- Only peel or chop vegetables just before they are to be used, for maximum retention of nutrients. If they have to be prepared in advance, store in an airtight container in the cold and dark.
- Do not overcook.
- Stir frying is a good way to cook vegetables, especially if an onion is used first. The high bioflavonoid content of onion reduces oxidation of the food as well as the oil so fewer undesirable free radicals are formed.
- Frozen vegetables often have a higher vitamin content than fresh ones, if they were frozen immediately after picking. Nutrient loss, especially vitamins B and C, is very fast on thawing however, so they should be cooked from frozen to minimise this.
- Vegetables are very valuable when eaten raw, as they contain live enzymes and vitamins which may be destroyed on cooking. Minerals are also lost in the water which goes down the sink. Cooking vegetables does not always cause vitamin loss. More beta-carotene, for example, is made available for use by the body when a carrot is cooked. It does not get thrown out in the cooking water as fat-soluble vitamins do not dissolve in water. This is good news; it increases our variety. Eat cooked and raw vegetables and enjoy them both.
- Although vegetables are used a lot by people on low-fat diets, it must be remembered that vitamins A, D and E are fat soluble and that beta-carotene from carrots needs a little fat or else most of it will be lost in the faeces. Eating nitrate-treated meats like ham with carrots will also cause loss of beta-carotene. However, beta-carotene will provide protection against the conversion of nitrate to nitrite in the gut, so if you must eat these treated meats, there is nothing for it but to have a double helping of carrots!

SALADS

Salads are important for healthy eating. Again, the crops are best taken when they are in season. In the winter there are still many alternatives to lettuce; red and white cabbage look very pretty, and Chinese leaves or chopped Brussels sprouts are also delicious. Be adventurous, try raw swede, raw beetroot, raw cauliflower, and even raw onions or leeks.

If your family will only eat salad with their favourite salad cream, try weaning them off it by putting natural yoghourt into a serving dish and adding the favourite salad cream, until you get the required taste. As the weeks go by, the yoghourt content goes up and the salad cream goes down.

Salad can also be used for starters. The French idea of *crudités* as a starter is a good one as it appears that eating raw vegetables before a meal offers some protection against the white blood cell destruction that occurs when cooked food is eaten.

FRUIT

Most of the comments about vegetables also apply to fruit.

They do not store for as long as root vegetables and the vitamin C content drops dramatically with storage and with thawing, if frozen. Fresh off a tree, the average orange has around 180 mg of vitamin C (some that have been stored in shops or in the house for months will have none at all). The acidity of most fruits is an important factor in the absorption of our minerals, iron in particular; it is therefore a good idea to take any mineral supplements with fruit or its juice. Be wary of aluminium cooking pans, and do not use them for stewing fruit; this includes tomatoes and other food like peppers which are really fruits, although we tend to use them as, and even sometimes call them, vegetables.

Fruit is our major source of bioflavonoids, sometimes known as vitamin P, which are valuable antioxidants. They work with vitamin C for maximum effect. Their major role is in strengthening the blood vessels, especially the little capillaries. A deficiency shows up as little thread veins in the skin. Bioflavonoids are especially rich in the pith of citrus fruits, which we often peel off. Vitamin C is quickly lost after chopping or grating the fruit or vegetables.

Fruit and vegetables are our main source of potassium. This mineral is essential for the heart and nervous system and it needs to be in balance with sodium for everything to work well. In this age of highly flavoured foods and liberally salted snacks, we need an awful lot of fruit to maintain the correct balance.

Dried fruit is an excellent source of potassium, as well as of other minerals like iron, copper and calcium. Unlike fresh fruit, they have usually been fully ripened before being picked and so have a good balance of nutrients. One problem, however, is that they are often coated with mineral oil to prevent sticking (see Chapter 14); such fruit needs thorough washing in hot water to remove this. Some are now treated with vegetable oil, which is much to be preferred as this does not tie up the fat-soluble vitamins A, D, E and K.

MEAT

Meat is a very good food, in moderation, but many adults eat too much of it and many children who need the protein more than adults, only eat the scrappy stuff in the chemically laden, highly processed varieties. Meat is high in methionine which requires vitamin B_6 for its utilisation. Diets high in meat content require extra vitamins A and B_6 to reduce the risk of atherosclerosis.

Primitive man ate the offal first when he made a kill and he gave the steak to his dogs. Today the offal is still the most nutritious part.

Meat should obviously be eaten fresh as it is a wonderful medium in which food poisoning bugs can grow. Fresh meat should be stored away from other foods in the fridge and should not be able to drip on to anything. Utensils used for raw meat should not be used for other ready-to-eat food. Barbecued meat is all right occasionally, but not as a regular meal as barbecueing increases the carcinogens. Adverse changes occur in any food which is overgrilled or burned.

Care must be taken that meat is adequately cooked, especially pork and chicken, and special care is needed if using a microwave oven. The use of clear film to cover food in the microwave is not as good as glass; high levels of a chemical called DEHA moves from this film into the fat parts of food with which it is in contact. Pre-chilled meat dishes are also risky.

There is no need to omit meat burgers from the diet, but try making your own with real meat. Minced meat in any form, burgers, pies, shepherds pie, etc., is invaluable for hiding high nutrient foods that the family will not otherwise eat. Sesame seeds, for example, have an excellent natural balance of calcium and magnesium, but are not part of a traditional British diet. These and pumpkin or sunflower seeds can be ground up and mixed in with the mince to give a nutrient-packed dish, excellent for young children and the elderly in particular.

If you wish to cook your own meat for cold meat, or perhaps you want to keep the fat for your own beef flavoured chips, remember to cook with onion. The high 'natural antibiotic' and bioflavonoid content of onion acts as a preservative and antioxidant. Onion or garlic will reduce the oxidation of oil, and so allow you to use it safely one more time.

FISH

Fish is not as popular as meat in this country, but nutritionally it is excellent. Many fish are only around 1 per cent fat, as compared with 33 per cent for meat, although this is not true of oily fish. These oily fish – the herring, mackerel, tuna, halibut, sardines, etc. – have their own plus factors for health, though, as they are high in the fats which offer protection from heart disease. Fish are a good source of vitamins and minerals; iodine, which is vital for thyroid function and so controls body metabolism, is especially high in seawater fish and hard to find elsewhere.

Fish is also high in choline, the B vitamin that gives fish their characteristic smell. Choline is a very important nutrient for boosting white blood cell numbers when necessary and also as a precursor for acetyl choline needed by the brain. It is not an old wives' tale that fish is good for the brain – it is.

The value of shellfish is a little controversial in these days of polluted waters, as they tend to accumulate pollutants readily. They are also high in cholesterol.

In general, though, fish is an ideal low-calorie high-nutrient low-fat real food. It yields important benefits to the immune system and health. Unfortunately children often do not want it, not so much because they do not like it, but because they cannot be fussed with the bones. Cartilaginous fish like skate are very easy to 'bone', and mackerel and flatfish like plaice and dab are also easy once the children have been shown the technique. Tinned fish are an even more valuable source of minerals as the bones can be eaten.

It is a pity to waste this excellent food because of the bones. Children are often delighted to make and eat fish cakes or fish burgers if the fish is boned for them first.

PULSES AND GRAINS

These are a favourite food for insects and do need to be stored in containers with tight-fitting lids. Heat dries and hardens them, so they are best not kept in a warm part of the kitchen. Sodium bicarbonate is often used in their cooking, especially if they have gone hard, but this does destroy much of their nutrient content, as well as increasing the levels of sodium in the body. Beans are at their best in September to October. After January, they become increasingly hard. Dusty pulses, grains and nuts should be avoided as they may be infected with a near invisible mould, and many of the substances produced by these moulds are toxic.

Many dried pulses should not be eaten raw as even the haricot bean, the type used in baked beans, contains antinutrients which could cause nausea, vomiting, diarrhoea and stomach cramps. These toxins are destroyed on cooking. Glycosides, like saponins, cause haemolysis of red blood cells; these chemicals are made inactive by soaking and by germination. If slow cookers are used for cooking, they should only be used on high settings, as low temperatures do not destroy harmful chemicals like phaeseolunatin and haemagglutinins.

Phosphorus is normally stored as phytic acid in grains, pulses, seeds and nuts. Phytic acid is essential for germination and so is used up during sprouting; it is also destroyed by acidic conditions, such as when yeast is used in bread making. Soaking beans or pulses in lemon juice or vitamin C also destroys this substance. Phytic acid is not good with every meal as it prevents absorption of our essential minerals. Again variety is important. The use of wholemeal flour in bread and white flour in some of the cakes is a good compromise. Enjoy a little of everything.

Wheat tends to be our staple grain, yet there are many others from which to choose. Try eating at least one different grain once a week; and by that I do not mean one helping of cornflakes or one bowl of porridge.

Rice

Rice needs to be washed five or six times until the water runs clear of starch. It is best not to stir it whilst cooking as this also releases starch, which makes the rice stick. The best results, nutritionally and visually, are obtained by adding rice to boiling water and boiling vigorously for two to three minutes. Next put on a tight lid and cook on a very low heat for around 20 minutes. Turn the heat off and leave until all the water is absorbed (8 oz of rice to 14 fl oz of water). Rice with beans gives protein which is sufficient in all amino acids.

Rice is a favourite food of the bacterium *Bacillus cereus*. It can withstand cooking for six hours, but it is not a problem in fresh cooked rice or cold rice stored below 2 °C. Do not, however, leave cooked rice at room temperature for a day or two as the bacillus could give your immune system an unwanted battle.

Barley

In the days of the Roman Empire, men were paid in barley. Today, many do not know what it looks like, although sprouted barley is essential for good beer. Barley, and malt extract derived from it, was used medicinally for respiratory infections.

Wholegrain barley needs about two hours to cook and it is often still very chewy; in contrast, pearl barley has had the outer layers removed, but is still nutritious. Do not buy it if the packet is dusty as it has probably had chalk added to make it look whiter. Always wash thoroughly.

Barley has a reasonable amount of potassium, but its 8 per cent protein is low in tryptophan and methionine.

Millet

Budgies may have small brains, but they know what is good for them. Just as eating bananas does not make you swing through the trees like a monkey, eating millet does not make you chirp like a bird or fly either; it may, however, help you to live longer, as the long-lived Hunza people eat it as their staple food. It is exceptionally high in potassium (ten times higher than pearl barley), and has twice as much magnesium as calcium, although it is quite high in both. Its limiting amino acid is lysine.

Millet needs at least four times its dry weight of liquid to cook. It can be used just like rice pudding or in savoury dishes.

Oats

Ask most people what they think of when you say the word oats, and the answer is either porridge or food for horses. It is true that oats is supposed to increase the friskiness of horses; it does this by increasing the excitability of muscles, which is brought about by an alkaloid in the pericarp of the oat grain which stimulates the motor ganglia of the nerves to the muscles.

Unfortunately, most of our oats are heat-treated. This destroys the enzyme, phytase, which would destroy the unwanted phytic acid. Treated oats as a major part of the diet could therefore leave you low on minerals. Oats are, nevertheless, a valuable food which is known to regulate body cholesterol levels and so is of special benefit to those with high cholesterol.

Steel-cut oatmeal is best as it has not been heat treated. This means that it can be soaked before it is cooked, the soaking allows the phytase time to destroy the phytic acid which robs the body of minerals. This type of oatmeal needs more cooking and does not keep as long; the heat treatment used in most of our oats, especially the instant variety, is to prevent the oil from going rancid so that it can be kept longer.

SEEDS

Sunflower seeds and oil are known to be important for their linoleic acid content. However, this varies depending on where the seeds come from; Russian sunflower seeds containing around 70 per cent linoleic acid are far superior to African sunflower seeds which contain only 20 per cent. Which is in the bottle on the supermarket shelf? British sunflowers stand a good chance of being high in this essential fatty acid as the content increases with the cooler climate. So grow your own, to eat at least!

Pumpkin seeds are rich in iron and zinc and have long been used to prevent prostate and bladder problems. Scientific research is now proving that there is a sound basis for using them for these problems.

Because of their relatively high fat content, both nuts and seeds should not be kept too long as they go rancid.

SNACKS

Snacks from bags, snacks from pots, snack meals – it's all big business. People often skip a meal in favour of several snacks, but to snack constantly all day is bad for the gut, especially when the snacks are high in fat and low in nutrients. High-fat foods, like chocolate and crisps (around 40 per cent fat) cause bile to be released into the gut, and a gut frequently soaked in bile is at increased risk of colon cancer.

The other problem with processed snacks and low-calorie diets is that they do not provide us with enough nutrients. Better snacks would be nuts, seeds, dried fruit, fresh fruit, grains and vegetables. Although vegetables for snacks might need to be prepared before going to work, they would still retain more micronutrients than a bar of chocolate. Fruit or vegetables dropped into a bowl containing three-quarters of a pint of water and half a teaspoon of vitamin C powder for a few seconds will not lose their colour, even after being cut. Homemade cakes and biscuits are far more nutritious than processed ones; they do not contain trans-fats, and favourite recipes can be made healthier by cutting down the usual fat and sugar content and raising the flour content.

Milk is also a very good snack food, especially for growing children and the elderly. Remember not to leave it in daylight as many vitamins are sensitive to light, especially A and D, which are important for bones and growth, and B_2. For those trying to give up packet bedtime drinks, molasses in hot milk is a very acceptable alternative; but you may only need to dip the teaspoon into the molasses and pull it out again – it can be very strong. It is also a good way of giving up flavoured sugar in milk. Molasses is a form of sugar, but so very little is needed that it in no way compares with two or three heaped teaspoons of malted milk or chocolate drink.

YOUR CHOICE

You can become accustomed to feeling a bit below par, come to accept this as the norm, without giving it much thought. There is a choice, however. Nutrients play a major part in rebuilding a flagging immune system. A variety of real nutrient-packed foods is an essential key to health, vitality and longevity. If we choose to use that key wisely and experiment a little, we may reap the benefits of becoming a chemist in the kitchen.

18
FOOD
PROCESSING

Man no longer fears a lot of his old enemies, like wild animals, or many of the deadly infectious diseases, such as smallpox. Now his most dangerous enemies are of his own creation. The immune system has many such enemies, the two over which we have the most control being the lack of nutrients in our food – nutrients needed to keep the immune system working properly – and the addition of substances to our food which will hinder the immune system's performance.

PESTICIDES – A HAZARD OR A HELP?

Man has always been possessive about his food – there have always been other creatures, ready, willing, able and hungry, to eat the fruit of his labours. Chemical pesticides were the answer to his dreams. Now he could spray his crops or land with some magic stuff and have it all to himself because nothing else wanted it. Wily worms wriggled off to pastures purer, and pests by the score packed their bags and left the poisons alone after they saw their fatal effect.

Man became very clever with these chemicals. There were fungicides for fungi, bactericides for bacteria, insecticides for insects, herbicides for weeds, miticides for mites, rodenticides for rodents, and fumigants which could tackle almost anything. There are now over 400 to choose from. But there is a lot of controversy as to whether they should be used at all.

Take insecticides for example. There are 800,000 different species of insect in the world and less than 1 per cent are harmful to plants, animals or humans; in fact, most of them help, by pollinating plants, by being part of the food chain for higher animals, by keeping other pests at bay and by helping with decomposition. Yet insecticides kill the lot, so disturbing the natural balance of things.

All of these affect people too. In 1971 nearly 40 people died in Honduras, and another 40 nearly died, when the group ate food which had been sprayed with an insecticide called Pallation. Many people died in Chiquinquira after eating bread made from poisoned flour; the flour had been transported in a truck which was carrying supplies of Parathion, one container had leaked and the flour had soaked it up. In another case, food was contaminated and people made ill after inhaling DDVP, a pesticide used on strips which were hung in rooms to kill flies. Through biological amplification, humans, at the top end of a long food chain, can take in greater and greater amounts of these pesticides; for example, in the USA breast-milk was found to contain unacceptable levels of DDT.

If we use chemicals to destroy the lives of other living things we must realise that these chemicals will also affect our bodies. The effects may be acute, as in the case of the people in Honduras, where they died relatively quickly, or they may be chronic, taking years to accumulate and to have their effect. Some pesticides like methyl bromide are poisonous for only a short time and then disperse, but they may adversely affect the food. Methyl bromide, for example, destroys some B vitamins, the poisonous effects of others like DDT, Aldrin, Dieldrin and Endrin last much longer, but they are usually cheaper.

Some pesticides act on contact, and some of those which are sprayed on to food can be washed or peeled off. Others are systemic; that is, they are taken into the fruit or plant and cannot be removed by washing or peeling. Many chemicals sprayed on food have similar properties. Alar, used to prevent apples falling from the tree, to promote uniform ripening and to get crisp apples, is a systemic chemical; it goes into the fruit. I came across a 1971 publication which carried Alar's warning label: 'Avoid breathing mist. May be harmful if swallowed. Toxic to fish. Do not graze animals on cover crops and apple orchards. Do not feed livestock apple pomace from Alar-treated apples.' In 1985 a US publication warned that it was very carcinogenic, only ethyl bromide rivalling it in its capacity to cause cancer, yet only at the end of 1989 did we see it banned in Britain.

It is difficult to ascertain the effects of these chemicals on people until they die, but post-mortem tests have shown high concentrations in fatty tissues of people who died of liver or central nervous diseases. Pesticides are being strongly linked with cancer and birth defects. The herbicide 2,4,5-T, put in the diet of rats and mice, led to abnormal offspring; yet 2,4,5-T was widely used as a defoliant in Vietnam and has been linked with a high rate of birth defects there. Most fungicides are known to be carcinogenic, yet they are sprayed on foods and even put into some breads.

Some of the effects of these toxic chemicals may be difficult to see.

Captan, for example, was thought to be non-toxic and vegetables were allowed residues of 100 ppm; but then it was found to have a disastrous effect on our DNA. It is not easy to see or feel genetic damage and it may take a generation or two before the effects become visible. Is it really worth risking genetic damage to get rid of weeds? Surely it would be better to use most of these pesticides only when absolutely necessary, not as a routine procedure, as many are used today? Unfortunately, a lot of money is spent on advertising and marketing these products.

Many such chemicals have been found to cause cancer, miscarriages, malformation, genetic damage or irritation after many years of use.

Furthermore, these pesticides also accumulate in the animals we eat. Most of them, the organochlorides in particular, build up in the fatty tissues, so cutting down on meat fat also cuts our pesticide consumption. Pesticides are not the only chemicals in our meat, however.

HORMONES AND ANTIBIOTICS

Feed additives like antibiotics, arsenicals, tranquillisers and hormones go in too.

Arsenic is fed as a supplement to many animals as it is necessary for growth, but it is important to get the dose right. Arsenic is an accumulative poison, so although the small dose in each mouthful of such meat may be insignificant, we do not want extra arsenic with every meal.

Tranquillisers also help to increase weight, not only because they make the animal move less, but also because they increase appetite. It is also thought that if we consume these tranquillisers via the food chain, they may slow down the speed with which we can carry out the chemical processes necessary for life, and this may be damaging in the long term.

Hormones cause our meat animals to put on weight, so increasing the financial gain. Of course, it will also give a hormone supplement to those who eat this meat if it is not withdrawn from the feed at least a week before slaughter. An excess of this hormone is certainly not desirable for men, and is not very good for women either as one of the theories on susceptibility to breast cancer is that it is associated with high levels of such female hormones. Many countries have banned the use in meat production of these hormones which are thought not only to cause breast cancer, but also to slow growth in children and to cause sterility or impotence in men.

The artificial growth of animals bred for meat has other side effects too. The carcass of an untreated free-grazing animal is 15 per cent protein and 5 per cent fat. (I often wonder if a human that sits around a lot and eats junk food could be compared in the same way with a 'free-range' individual living on as additive-free a diet as he can manage? Would we get leaner without even dieting if we did not have to ingest all those additives? Perhaps we should all start counting chemicals instead of calories.)

FERTILISERS

Fertilisers are necessary to put nutrients back into the soil which crops have taken out. It is important that all nutrients be put back into the soil; a recycling of our resources is an important link in the life cycles that perpetuate good health. Unfortunately, we no longer use natural methods of recycling, as cheap synthetic nitrogen fertilisers visibly do the trick. Or do they?

They make crops grow well, but sadly the crops do not have the same vitamin and mineral content as crops grown on a well-balanced nutrient-rich soil. Not only are they vitamin and mineral deficient; they often have very high nitrate levels as well.

High nitrate intake is linked with cancer, in particular gut and bladder cancers. It is not the nitrate that causes the problem so much as the nitrites which are formed from it. Nitrites are used in cured meats, where they prevent the growth of the bug which causes botulism; and they are also found in food which is stale or has been stored badly.

Bugs that turn nitrates into nitrites are common in babies' stomachs. In areas where nitrates used in farming have caused high levels of nitrates in the water, there were 'blue baby' problems. Now, in such areas, water with lower levels of nitrate has to be supplied for babies.

Lettuce, tomatoes and various other fruits and vegetables are grown under glass and with high concentrations of nitrate, sometimes even without soil. The nutrients supplied by these plants are far less than those grown under normal conditions, while the nitrate levels are artificially high. It is questionable whether these foods are worth eating, but how does the consumer know how his lettuce was grown? It is usually safer to buy food which is in season as it is less likely to have been artificially reared.

Nitrosamines are potent carcinogens. They are found at higher levels in the bodies of tobacco smokers. They are also formed in the presence of combined nitrite and protein derivatives. Vitamin C and E prevent their formation, as do acid conditions, but stomach acidity is often poor in infants and the elderly, so these are particularly vulnerable to damage by these chemicals. Vitamins C and E levels are lower in forced foods and in stored foods, and may even be removed in processed foods, so they are often deficient at a time when we need more.

FOOD IRRADIATION

Good food does not need to be irradiated. Good food should go bad. This is how we know that it is no longer fit to eat and could harm us. Bad food could introduce bugs or chemicals that our immune systems would have to work hard to get rid of. Irradiation will not improve the food. It will, however, destroy some of the nutrients, especially vitamins C, B_1, B_2, B_6, A, E, folic acid, cysteine and the essential fatty acids, i.e. the type of fat that we are encouraged to eat for health.

Irradiation will also mean that food which has started to go bad will miraculously look good again at the wave of a cobalt or caesium wand. The salmonella bug is often destroyed, if the dosage is high enough and the strain has not become resistant, but the bug which causes botulism (*Clostridium botulinum*) and many other viruses are not completely destroyed by this process. Clostridium spores are resistant and can grow again, and toxic chemicals produced by these bugs are not destroyed either. In other words, if your meat or whatever has been contaminated by clostridium and been renovated (a charming and respectable name for making old bad food look as fresh as new), the poison already in the food could make you seriously ill or even cause death.

A study on malnourished Indian children whose diet included 50 per cent irradiated food showed that they developed abnormal white blood cells with multiple chromosomes. The study was stopped immediately and the children's cells returned to normal. A similar experiment was continued on rats and these soon showed malformations in offspring.

The vast majority of the population do not need sterilised food. Our guts need many of the good bacteria in food in order to remain clean and healthy – they are our internal housekeepers. Irradiation seems to be an unwanted, unnecessary and potentially dangerous process. No one knows the damage that totally new radiolytic products will do to our bodies and immune systems. Should we really risk genetic damage on a large scale?

It is true that all irradiated foods will legally have to be marked as such, but will it? How can you tell if it has been renovated or not, if no one wants to tell you? As a process, it is useful for preparing food for severely immune suppressed patients who need food which has no bugs in it at all. It could also be useful for astronauts; in years to come we may be happy to have full board when going on that holiday to the moon, but in the meantime there are too many unanswered questions about the effect this process will have on our health to use it on our daily food.

DEVALUATION OF FOOD

There are nearly 4,000 permitted additives that can be used in our food, and it is estimated that 75 per cent of the average diet in this country is made up of processed food. As a lot of people try to avoid processed food most of the time, others must be eating a lot more than this.

We use additives to make food look and taste better, especially if it is of poor quality and flavour in the first place. Additives also make food easier for the manufacturer to work with, convenient for the consumer to use, fast to prepare at home and able to last longer.

All 4,000 additives do the job they were intended to do very well, but what else do they do? What other effects do they have on our bodies? Most of all, what effect do they have in combination? An average processed meal may contain 10 or 20 different added chemicals.

Flavours

Although many additives are now labelled with E numbers (a European Community designed coding to help identify the additives), 3,500 of those 4,000 additives are flavours and there is no law which makes manufacturers tell us what those flavours are.

Flavours are very useful, allowing fat, salt, sugar and starch to form the basic ingredients for anything from savoury dishes to soups and desserts, these same ingredients being altered by flavours to give the required dish. Other additives make the colour and texture right. A strawberry-flavoured dessert may have never seen a strawberry, but if it's coloured pink and has added strawberry flavour, it is accepted as such by the consumer. In reality, though, a processed food diet that may seem very varied thanks to the expensive marketing, exotic names and chemical cocktails may actually be a very bland, unbalanced, monotonous, low-nutrient and unhealthy diet.

When food is preserved, much of its flavour is lost. Flavours and flavour enhancers are added to disguise this and to make us think that the product is good food. Many flavours and flavour enhancers that have been used for years have now been withdrawn as they are found to have adverse effects on animals and humans. Monosodium glutamate, for example, has long been used without restriction, but because it has been found to cause brain damage in baby mice it is now banned from baby foods, even though many infants eat the highly flavoured snacks which do contain this additive. Safrole and one of the artificial vanilla flavours called coumarin are now thought to be carcinogenic. How many more will join the list? These substances are not food, so why are they permitted to contaminate our food when they could damage our health?

Real food tastes good and has an added bonus – it does you some good. Poor quality stale food, however, needs added flavours and usually costs a lot more, both in money and calories.

Colours
Many foods lose colour in processing, so colours are used to replace them, over 75 per cent of these being synthetic dyes usually derived from coal tar. They are now often banned as they are becoming notorious for causing cancer and for their effect on children's behaviour. (Many colours like tartrazine are avoided by careful mothers.) Several red and yellow dyes, in particular, have been found to be carcinogenic and one, Citrus Red, was used to colour the skins of oranges – which, of course, do not have to be labelled.

Preservatives
These, at least, fulfil a need. If food is processed or handled a lot, it may need a preservative to keep down the bug content, but the use of many preservatives is abused. Some people died after high levels of sodium nitrate were added to fish that had already gone bad, in an attempt to make the fish saleable. If a large dose can have such an effect, what effects do lots of smaller ones have? Nitrates in the diet need to be kept down, not constantly incremented.

Sulphur dioxide is another toxic chemical when used in excess. It bleaches rot spots in fruit to make it look good, but it forms sulphuric acid and destroys B vitamins. It is often used for dried fruit, so read the label; much of it can be washed off. Sugar and salt are also used as preservatives, and are fine in moderation.

Our natural antioxidants are vitamin C in our watery tissues and fluids and vitamin E in our fatty parts, but they are often destroyed or taken out during processing, artificial preservatives then being added. NDGA (nor-dihydrogauiaretic acid) was used for years before it was shown to have adverse effects on the immune system, causing lesions in the lymph nodes, and haemorrhages. BHT (butylated hydroxytoluene) and BHA (butylated hydro-oxyanisole) are preservatives restricted in many countries.

Sweeteners
Artificial sweeteners are cheaper than sugar, but may cost a lot in other ways. Cyclamates were banned in many countries as they were thought to be a danger if consumed regularly for long periods. Saccharin, too, is suspected to be carcinogenic, if taken regularly over long periods.

Even aspartame, a relatively new sweetener made from the amino acids aspartic acid and phenylalanine, is not without its problems; some individuals especially those with phenylketonuria are sensitive to it. It can put the amino acid pool out of balance if taken in excess and it is broken down into methanol, which is transformed into formaldehyde, the stuff used to preserve laboratory specimens. Are we using so many added artificial preservatives that we are being pickled from the inside? On top of this, cancer cells that cause melanoma love phenylalanine. One has to question the wisdom of sitting for too many hours in the sun sipping vast quantities of diet soft drinks, with or without the alcohol.

Other chemicals
Emulsifiers are so good at doing their job that, unfortunately, they continue to do it in the body and increase the chances of retaining unwanted chemicals like pesticides.

Chemical sequestrants are added to foods to make some of the less desirable metals in the food harmless. They do this by chemically locking them up so that they cannot be used. Unfortunately, these continue to work in the body and tie up essential cobalt, iron, copper and zinc.

CONCLUSION

The human body cannot make its own food from the elements. It needs to eat to live. It breaks down pre-made plant or animal material and rebuilds this into its own shape and form. It uses food to build and arm an immune army.

We can sabotage, confuse and hinder this army by giving it unknown chemicals disguised as food. Chemically laden nutrient-free foods will not promote health and can cause temporary or permanent illness, and even premature death.

We need to take a long look at the production and consumption of our food. It is the stuff that life is made of and, although we should be able to enjoy it and make money from producing it, the primary concerns must be to provide food which gives health rather than wealth; which provides essential nutrients in quantities that you can measure rather than concentrating on empty calories merely to provide gastronomic pleasure.

19
WATER

Man, complex though he is, is over 70 per cent water, and can only live for three or four days without this precious resource.

Water is vital for all life on earth, flowing, not only through our streams and rivers, but also through the sap of trees and plants and through our veins and arteries. Most living things have a high water content, ranging from the desert rat, which is around a mere 65 per cent water, to apples and earthworms which are about 80 per cent. Tomatoes and jellyfish are nearer 95 per cent water.

Water is used for many life processes, but most especially for internal cleansing and feeding. All the poisons and waste accumulated in the body are excreted in solution, be it tears, sweat or urine, and water is needed to extract many nutrients from food. Water is in many ways a forgotten nutrient for animals, although we still recognise it as a major nutrient in plants. We take it for granted.

Every water molecule is made up of one oxygen atom and two hydrogen atoms – hence its chemical symbol H_2O. It is rarely found in the absolutely pure state, as water's excellent dissolving powers means that it readily takes up other substances. The sea is usually alkaline, with a pH around 8, because of the salts dissolved in it. Our sweat and urine are preferably acid, due to the different substances dissolved in them which are necessary to deter bacterial growth.

The marvellous dissolving ability of water is essential for many biological systems, but we tend to abuse its cleaning power.

POLLUTION OF WATER

Man has always needed to live near water. If his water source became unacceptable, he would move on to another. After a few years, bacteria would have worked on the unacceptable source, broken down all the organic matter and made it fit to live next to and use once again. Water pollution has always been a problem, but the pollution used to be biodegradable.

Nowadays, however, we pollute with lead, aluminium, mercury, glass, plastics, pesticides, fertilisers, detergents, medicines, oil and all sorts of other rubbish that these bacteria do not fancy eating. And who can blame them? We all play a part in polluting the water and can all help to reduce the problem.

Many of man's domestic activities require detergents. Whilst these products do the job that they were developed to do very well, making everything cleaner than clean and whiter than white, they also make the water dirty.

Furthermore, many medicines, from antibiotics to tranquillisers and the pill, go down the sink or the loo every day. These are not easily removed from the water when it is recycled. Some of these medicinal drugs taken will inevitably pass into the water supply after their voyage through the body, but we can all help to reduce our water pollution by at least returning unwanted medicines to the chemist.

We can also use low-phosphate detergents. Algae love phosphates and so grow profusely in our freshwater lakes and reservoirs when phosphates are present. Their death and decomposition use up oxygen in the water and their large numbers reduce the available light, so that plants and animals beneath cannot breathe or feed. The food chain breaks down and eventually the river or lake dies.

The process by which a youthful water source matures, ages and eventually dies is known as eutrophication. By our thoughtless and selfish actions, we have accelerated the aging process of many of our beautiful lakes by tens of thousands of years.

It is not only the trees that we can see that we are destroying, but also those that live beneath the sea. Underwater kelp forests have been wiped out, but because we cannot see this for ourselves, we do not think of the consequences. As the oceanic plant life produces about 60 per cent of the world's newly released oxygen every year, the loss of these forests affects us directly. We cannot afford to lose them; we must appreciate their value and protect them, before it is too late to reverse their destruction.

LOOKING AFTER OUR WATER

Water authorities have the job of looking after our water and making it fit to drink. Some have a more difficult job than others, depending on the quality of the raw water which they have to treat. Some waters flowing through peat will be very acidic to start with and may well have high aluminium levels. Others may have high nitrate levels, because they flow through farming areas. Some have high levels of lead, etc.

Like any other businessmen, the authorities are concerned about what the consumer wants. We therefore need to be aware of what is added to the water and what it naturally contains, and to ask questions if we feel something is not right.

Most people, and hence many water authorities, are concerned mainly about the look and taste of the water. We should remember our most important need for water; it is to drink. It is much more important to have water which is high in the minerals that we need for health, and low in any toxic materials, than it is to have water which looks like Perrier, and does not leave scale or scum in the kettle or round the loo.

Chlorination

Since the introduction of water treatment plants in this country, we rarely have problems with waterborne diseases, and certainly not from our tapwater. This is largely due to chlorination of our water supplies. There is some concern over the possible carcinogenic properties of trihalomethanes (a byproduct of water treated with chlorine), but the risk is small in comparison with drinking untreated water which could cause disease. It is preferable to use chlorine rather than nothing as long as water authorities do this responsibly and do not overdose our water supplies. Trihalomethane levels tend to be higher in the east of England.

Iron and manganese

Although many authorities are bothered with high iron and manganese levels, this is mainly for cosmetic reasons. Actually, a little more iron and manganese would be good for most of us; both these elements are essential for a healthy, active immune system, and deficiency is common. If you live in a high iron or manganese area, try to forget that you cannot get your washing whiter than white (after all, neither can the person next door), and just think how much good these two minerals are doing for your immune system.

Calcium and magnesium

These are two more 'contaminants' of pure water that people seem to want to get rid of, principally because they shorten the life of kettles, washing machines and water heating systems. These elements may clog up electrical gadgets, but a shortage of them in the human body most definitely shortens healthy active life. Which life is more important to you, yours or that of your kettle?

Hard water areas have much higher levels of calcium and magnesium than soft water areas, and consumption of hard water has long been associated with the prevention of heart disease. This may be due to the magnesium content, as magnesium deficiency is very common in this country (along with heart disease); some heart flutters or arrhythmias are merely due to a magnesium deficiency, and can be corrected by magnesium supplementation. The calcium in hard water also helps keep blood calcium levels up, so reducing the body's need to pull calcium out of the bones, and reducing many of the age-related bone problems.

Calcium and magnesium together are wonderful chemical buffers and it has been shown that the toxic effects of antinutrients like lead and aluminium are far greater in their absence.

Nitrates
We still use a lot of nitrate fertilisers, and leached water which drains through this treated soil can have quite high nitrate levels, depending on the type of rock and soil.

Many of our water sources are from underground aquifers, and the water in these may date back 30 or more years to a time before the large-scale use of these fertilisers. But nitrate levels are rising, and so are the number of sources which exceed the acceptable, though not necessarily desirable, level of 50 mg/litre. This trend is worrying, because even if we halved the use of nitrogen fertilisers now, levels could still rise for the next 30 or so years. Nitrate is notoriously difficult to get out of water and the treatment is quite expensive. In excess, it does have an adverse effect on our health, as has been seen in Chapter 18.

FILTERED AND BOTTLED WATER

It is always wise to find out if there is anything in the local water which needs to be removed, and which a filter can remove, before purchasing one. If the water is not high in lead or copper or other undesirable elements, it is probably not worth bothering. Nitrates are not removed by most filters.

Most water filters need very frequent changing in hard water areas, because they remove calcium from water and this quickly clogs up the filter.

Although filters remove chlorine, leaving tap water to stand or boiling it will also remove the free chlorine.

So, is it worth buying bottled water? The answer is that it depends on why you are buying it. If you like the fizz of sparkling waters, then it is worth buying what you like. If, however, you are buying it because you think it is 'cleaner' than tap water, it is probably not worth it as the bacteriological count is often higher than tap water in this country. Filter water may be even worse if the filter has not been changed often enough, as bacteria grow on the nutrients in the filter. Bottled water does not contain pathogenic (harmful) bacteria, but neither does tap water in Britain. Filters, however, will grow whatever bugs are around and, in unhygienic surroundings, may grow disease-causing bugs.

Sparkling waters contain less bacteria than still water. This could be due to the addition of carbon dioxide (which gives it the fizz) or to its lower oxygen content. Water is an important source of oxygen for our cells, and oxygen tends to be removed by carbonation and boiling; so we should not drink these types of water exclusively.

Although it is called mineral water, the mineral content of bottled water is often very low; it would take a lot of this water to 'supplement the diet'. Safeway Braeuisge Spring is quite high in fluoride and is not your best choice if you are trying to avoid this, while the French Badoit and Sainsbury's Scottish Spring are rather higher in sodium than all the others and should be avoided if you are trying to stick to a low-sodium diet.

Although all of the mineral waters tested had less than half the nitrate of high-nitrate tap water, many were higher than low-nitrate areas. If you live in an area where nitrate levels are high, it may be worth buying bottled water.

Bottled water does not keep once opened; it goes off, so bottled (or filtered) water should be boiled first if used for baby food or drink.

Labelling

The labelling laws are not very specific on any drink in this country. Wines and beers are classic examples of manufacturers getting away with putting all sorts of non-food materials into their products because they do not have to state their ingredients like food manufacturers have to do. All drinks suffer from the labelling loophole, although it would be very helpful to the consumer if they did display a contents list. It is not an imposition; if manufacturers wish us to consume their products, we have a right to know what is in them.

Unfortunately, labelling for bottled water is really only to promote advertising and sales. Labels that say 'pure' mean nothing. Pure water never exists naturally, so leave pure water for the fairies to bathe in, we want some nutritional mineral 'contaminants'. Also ignore labels that offer calorie-free water; all water, including tap water, is calorie free.

WATER AS A NUTRIENT

The demand for water will continue to increase with increasing population and increasing technological advances, but how does it affect us and our health?

The body of an average man can contain as much as 45 litres of water. We lose and replace water every day. Just resting for a day in our temperate climate, we would expect to lose 1 litre of water. If we were in the tropics, it could be a litre and a half.

Even fasting, we would use around a third of a litre in the chemical processes of oxidising stored carbohydrates and fats. Eating, we would use more. Feeding and working hard manually in the heat could cause a loss of around 4.5 litres of water. Some would also be lost flushing the kidneys. We use water as a chemical for most of our metabolic processes, from building ourselves up to breaking down our food. Physically, we use it as a lubricant so that we can move.

Different people have different water contents, ranging from 56 to 80 per cent. It has been shown that as we age we lose our thirst, our bodies dry out a little and physical shrinking can begin. Organs get slightly smaller and so does the brain; sometimes air pockets are formed in the skull. But it has been shown that these early signs of senility can be reversed by drinking the correct amount of water. In other words, we can age our brains and bodies prematurely by not drinking enough water.

We replace our own water loss every day and build this 'new' water into our tissues. Of course, our bodies and health are bound to be adversely affected if we continuously drink water laced with medicinal drugs, pesticides, hormones, detergents, fertilisers, radioactive waste, toxic chemicals and various other combinations of poisons. The immune system has to deal with all of these contaminants, many of which it does not recognise and does not know what to do with. So it tries to tidy them away somewhere. The bones, joints, tissues or brain are common storage depots.

Many of these contaminants are cumulative. For example, arsenic, aluminium and lead build up year after year; by middle age the lead or aluminium in the knees or brain could have accumulated enough to start letting you know about their presence. Then the creaks and groans and memory slips begin. The effects of some of these antinutrient contaminants will be dealt with in the next chapter.

It is in all of our interests to protect our water. It constitutes, after all, around 70 per cent of all of us. Be clean, be green and take an interest in your local water – it is the future you.

20
ANTINUTRIENTS

Common salt is a compound, sodium chloride. The compound is made up of two different elements, sodium and chlorine. Some elements like sodium, calcium, magnesium, iron, etc., serve as nutrients to the body. They are necessary, either to build the body or for carrying out some of the body's chemical reactions.

Elements like lead, mercury, cadmium and aluminium do not have any known useful function in the body. In fact, not only are they not nutrients, they positively hinder natural body function. Fluorine is another element which can cause havoc and destruction in the body, although it has been claimed to have a beneficial effect on teeth. Some of us would put fluorine and its compounds in the antinutrient list above, others would put it along with arsenic in that grey area bordering on antinutrients.

Antinutrients interfere with a lot of the body's essential chemistry; the immune system is only one affected part, although a very critical one. Minimising antinutrient intake can do a lot to improve health.

WHY FIGHT FLUORIDE?

Kilsilcaoern, in Turkey, is the real-life opposite of Shangri-la. Far from being a place of eternal youth, it is a place where people age faster than their years. It is nicknamed *Das Dorf der Jungen Greise* (or the village of old young people).

Children and animals have brown teeth; adults rarely have any. Stillbirths are very common, as are four-month miscarriages. Walking is painful and bones are twisted before the age of 30, with every inhabitant of the village suffering from a bone disease which causes thickening of the bones. Muscles are weak, skin is wrinkled. It is not surprising that most of the people suffer from depression. They do not know why they are like this whilst people in other distant villages are not. The fluoride content of their water is given as 5.4 parts per million. Although the most severely afflicted, they are not alone in their symptoms; people in Acquaviva Platani in Sicily share their problems, as do those in the Dharwar district in Karnataka, and other small areas of India.

There are many reports of fluoride aggravating arthritis and other bone disorders in western countries, but here we are well fed. In some of the poor Indian villages the people do not have the nutrients to build up what fluoride has broken down. It has since been shown that fluoride at levels as low as one part per million causes breakdown of collagen – around a third of our body protein is collagen. With collagen building-blocks we build skin, muscle, cartilage and bone. Here in the west we can rebuild the damage: the malnourished people in India and Turkey cannot. However, what is the point of causing this destruction in the first place, and possibly hastening premature aging, if it is not necessary?

Fluorine comprises about 0.004 per cent of body weight, but is regarded as poisonous if more than 5 grams are present in the body. The *Merck Index* lists it as below:

Human Toxicity: Severe symptoms from ingestion of less than 1 gram, death from 5 to 10 grams. SUBLETHAL: Nausea, vomiting, abdominal distress, diarrhoea, stupor, weakness. LETHAL: Muscular weakness, tremors, convulsions, respiratory and cardiac failure, death. CHRONIC: Mottling of tooth enamel, osteosclerosis. Use: As insecticide, particulaly for roaches and ants, in other pesticide formulations.

Toothpaste

We are becoming much too lax with fluoride. Advertising makes it into a completely safe, beneficial chemical which, like fairy dust spread over a toothbrush wand, will magic perfect teeth, but we need to realise the dangers of fluoride.

Fluoride toothpaste contains around 1,000 parts per million fluoride. One tube (7 oz) contains enough fluoride to kill a small child of up to 20 lb if he ate the lot in one go.

Artificial fluoridation of water has been banned in Sweden, and scientists there issue a warning to parents that, if they live in naturally high fluoride areas, pre-school children should only be allowed to brush their teeth with fluoridated toothpaste once a day, using only a pea-sized amount of toothpaste.

Fluoride tablets

We are led to believe that fluoride tablets are only beneficial, but this is far from the case. Evidence on the ability of fluoride to strengthen teeth is very contradictory. If you choose to take fluoride tablets, they should, like any other tablets, be kept under lock and key, safely away from young children.

Jason Burton died five days after lapsing into a coma. His mother left the toddler having an afternoon sleep, but he woke up and she found him sitting on the floor with the bottle of fluoride tablets. Jason had eaten six in one go, but he had had one every day since his first birthday and his mother had taken them when she was pregnant. It was a high price to pay for teeth.

Fluoride sensitivity

It is worth noting that some people are more sensitive to fluoride than others, children in particular. It is best to remove all fluoride toothpaste, rinses and tablets if your child has been using them and frequently has tummy aches, is pale and tired, perhaps with a poor appetite and frequent sickness.

Fluoride should not be added to water supplies; it is simply not true to say that 1 mg/litre of fluoride in water is 'safe' – so much depends on how much water you drink daily.

- The actual dosage obtained varies. If you drink 1 litre of water per day your dose from this is 1 mg; if you drink 6 litres per day, your dose is 6 mg.
- Water may not be your only source. The average diet contains about 1.3 mg of fluoride per day.

Everyone has to drink water and it is wrong to contaminate it with a potential poison when it is not necessary for improving the water. It removes freedom of choice about consuming such a controversial chemical.

Fluoride reduces immune power

Altering the code

As you already know, the immune system recognises foreign organisms or particles by an amino acid code. It rejects all codes it does not recognise. Our dead and damaged cells will also have a damaged code and so will be disposed of. Similarly, the immune army recognises sequences of amino acids which represent self and leaves them alone.

Proteins are made up of amino acids, and it has been found that fluoride interferes with the bonds that hold our proteins in the correct shape. In altering the shape of the body's own proteins, fluoride could alter the body's response to itself and cause auto-immune and/or allergy problems.

Slowing down the immune system
White blood cells travel around the body in the blood and lymph. When they find something wrong, they have to move towards it by a chemical attraction in order to destroy it. It has been found that white blood cells from people living in fluoridated areas are much slower at moving towards the enemy; after exposure to 0.1 mg/litre of fluoride for six hours, migration of human white blood cells is reduced by a fifth, and the ability of white cells to move in this way decreases with an increase in fluoride.

Decreasing the ability to destroy
Other studies show that one part per million of fluoride increases the body's cyclic AMP (adenosine monophosphate), a substance which reduces the white cell's ability to destroy foreign invaders by phagocytosis.

Super-oxygen
Fluoride confuses white blood cells by getting them to produce superoxide, a toxic oxygen molecule, when they do not need to and by preventing them from doing so when they actually do need to destroy a germ with superoxide. The superoxide produced when not needed could overspill into the blood or lymph and cause tissue damage.

Protein destruction
Fluoride disrupts body protein by breaking down collagen and interfering with its repair, tending to make it uneven. Because of this, it can disrupt any part of us that contains protein. The muscles are particularly susceptible. Athletes need to be careful of an excess as they could increase their chances of weakened muscles and torn ligaments or tendons.

Fluoride can also cause mineralisation in tissues which should not be mineralised: scleroderma, or calcification of skin collagen, is one example; hardening of the arteries is another. Fluoride may be a contributory factor to both. Joints may exhibit mineralisation and tend to become solid; the spine is also particularly susceptible to fluoride-induced ragged bony outgrowths.

Furthermore, fluoride is a potent inhibitor of enzymes. The enzyme which is needed to repair our genetic material can be slowed down considerably by fluoride. Weight loss can be impaired, as one part in 15 million of fluoride will reduce the effectiveness of lipase (a fat splitting enzyme) by 50 per cent.

Hormones are also affected; for example, thyroxin, the thyroid hormone, production decreases (thyroxin helps the body to burn fuel and to give energy).

MERCURY

Mercury and the immune system

Having an excess of mercury in the body can definitely adversely affect your ability to fight off infections, as it reduces both the B and the T lymphocytes. Not only does it reduce their numbers, but it also slows down the movement of T lymphocytes towards their prey, and attacks sulphur–hydrogen links which hold antibodies together.

Furthermore, it has been shown that mercury can alter the genetic material in lymphocytes. Lymphocytes have genetic material that is 'programmed' to tell them which bits belong to you and which bits are foreign and do not. If the 'programming' is changed by mercury there may be a number of results. Lymphocytes may no longer recognise self and could start attacking vital bits, as in autoimmune diseases. Secondly, in studies of animals with mercury poisoning, their systems started making antibodies to their own poisoned white cells. Thirdly, it could increase the incidence of allergy by recognising something like egg, for example, which is really harmless, and treat it as if it were an enemy, or finally it could totally ignore a real enemy.

Other effects

Favourite sites for the accumulation of mercury are the red blood cells, kidneys, heart, lungs and brain, but it is not really fussy and once it is in the system it can go almost anywhere. It can cross the blood-brain barrier; it then affects the brain and nervous system (hence madness, behavioural and psychological problems). It can be stored in our fat, and can travel in the lymph as well as the blood. It damages the sensory organs; vision becomes much narrower and deafness is common. And it can affect the cardiovascular and endocrine (hormone) systems.

Love for sulphur

Because mercury has a special attraction for sulphur-to-hydrogen (S–H) bonds, anything with such bonds is disrupted by its presence.
- Haemoglobin is very rich in these bonds, so red blood cells are the prize targets. The blood can even be prevented from clotting properly.

- Acetyl choline, a neurotransmitter, has these bonds, and its disruption affects heart muscle and the memory.
- Myosin, a muscle protein, has the bonds and so all muscle, including the heart, can be affected.

Enzymes

Without enzymes our body chemistry would be so slow that we would not survive; enzymes are necessary to speed up all of the chemical processes needed for survival. We have hundreds of enzymes in the body and many of them have the S–H bond, because they contain the amino acid cysteine. Cysteine is also found in ribosomes (sites of protein synthesis in the cells), in antibodies and in hormones; for example, the hormone insulin is a vulnerable one – by disrupting insulin mercury interferes with our blood sugar levels and hence lowers our energy levels. Energy is also lowered because mercury upsets two of our most important energy-producing enzymes – acetyl and succinyl CoA.

Anti-oxidant enzymes like superoxide dismutase and glutathione peroxide are also affected, and this can increase the risk of cancers and heart disease from free radical damage.

Mercury accidents

Grains

Grains are often treated with an anti-mildew spray when they are to be stored and later used as seed. The spray often contains mercury, so grains like this should not be used for food. However, occasionally accidents happen.

One such accident happened in Iraq in 1972, when 459 people died and 6,350 were hospitalised, all with methyl mercury poisoning. This was not the first incident in Iraq, although it was the worst; similar accidents had happened in 1956 and 1960.

Fish

Around 50 people were killed and many unborn babies died or suffered badly with an incident related to contaminated fish in Japan. An irresponsible plastics factory discharged mercury-containing waste into the Minamata River.

Mercury, unfortunately, is one of the poisons which can cross the placental barrier (one of the reasons why pregnant mums are now advised to wait until after the baby's birth to have amalgam fillings put in or removed) and many of the pregnant mums were badly affected by the mercury in the fish. Many miscarried and others had unhealthy babies.

Poisoned slimmer
In the 1970s there was a poison scare in the United States. Swordfish were said to contain very large amounts of mercury, but the warning came too late for one lady who had decided to slim by going on a swordfish diet. As this was all she had eaten for a few weeks, she became very ill. (This also serves to highlight the dangers of silly diets that revolve around eating only one or two foods.)

Hair analysis
Hair analysis is now regarded as reliable for toxic metals (although you should be very sceptical of claims that it can detect allergies, etc.). Some of Sir Isaac Newton's hair was tested in this way quite recently, to try and explain a period of very irrational behaviour he went through in the middle of his brilliant career. The diary that he had kept just previous to his madness listed his experiments, which were all with quicksilver (the common name for mercury at the time). He had inhaled the vapours during his experiments, and his hair was found to contain 197 ppm, as compared to 5 ppm in normal hair. He became a recluse for a while to get over his problem, before returning to his work, although he never regained his former brilliance. It is fortunate that mercury does eventually find its way out of the body, unlike some poisons.

Should you find high mercury levels in a hair analysis, try to avoid further contamination and increase protective foods and supplements, as described at the end of this section.

Sources of mercury

Mercury in medicine
Mercury products have been used in medicine since before the time of Christ, probably because it was noticed that it killed anything from bugs to man – the trick was getting the dose right. It first became really famous as a drug against syphilis at a time when there was no other cure.

It has long been used with other metals in dentistry, as amalgam fillings. Unfortunately evidence now suggests that some linings leak and allow mercury through the pulp of the tooth into the tissues and blood. Some mercury may be released on chewing, or be vaporised when we drink hot beverages, eat hot food or smoke. Streptococci in the dental plaque and throat add to the release of mercury. It is worth trying not to swallow bits of filling when it is removed or put in.

Some suppositories for haemorrhoids, some diuretics, laxatives, disinfectants and psoriasis creams still contain mercury.

Food sources of mercury
The food sources are mainly fish, although ocean fish suffer less with this problem than freshwater fish and shellfish in or near an estuary. This is because high mercury levels are found in estuarine waters, due to man's constant chemical dumping in rivers and along coastlines.

Vegetables may be contaminated with it if they have been fertilised with sewage sludge.

Industrial sources
- A lot of mercury is released into the environment in the process of making chlorine.
- Agriculture uses mercury in antimildew sprays.
- Burning coal releases a lot of mercury vapour into the air.
- Mercury compounds are used in the production of plastics, fireworks and explosives.
- Fur processing requires the use of mercury; this is what made Alice in Wonderland's famous Mad Hatter mad. Those in the fur hat trade were known to develop madness after years of working in an atmosphere contaminated with mercury.

Bacterial intervention
Oral doses of mercury are usually less toxic than if it is inhaled, but nevertheless common bugs like *E. coli*, staphylococci, streptococci and yeasts will methylate the mercury for you and render it more toxic and absorbable. Streps are quite common in the mouth and throat, so acting on the mercury on its way down.
- The acidophilus bugs found in yoghourt are very discerning and help to excrete mercury quickly, thus protecting us from mercury poisoning.

Protective nutrients
- vitamin C is good at reducing the harmful effects of most heavy metals. If hair analysis shows high mercury levels, vitamin C in a three-to-one ratio with cysteine is a good supplement.
- Selenium is especially protective because it is part of some

enzymes which get rid of the free radicals which mercury causes.

- Vitamin E is useful in helping selenium, calcium and magnesium to provide protection against any heavy metal or aluminium absorption.
- Pectin and alginate will offer some protection against inorganic mercury.

LEAD

Lead is a systemic poison; that is, it accumulates in the body, eventually producing problems that develop slowly.

Lead has been recognised as a powerful poison since early civilisation. It has even been postulated that it was lead poisoning that caused the fall of the Roman Empire. The Romans used pewter (lead and tin) plates, mugs, cooking pots and utensils, and their wine was stored in pewter casks. Ancient writings show that many individuals suffered with behavioural and physical problems that we now associate with lead poisoning. The more they ate and drank, the more lead was leached out of their utensils into their food and drink and then into their bones and brains.

Bodies of those who died on the Franklin Arctic expedition in search of the Northwest Passage, were found to contain high levels of lead. So it may not have been just the extreme conditions which overcame them, but also the lead solder in their tins of food. (Ironically, lead solder was prohibited from tins containing pet food before it was banned from use on tins containing food for human consumption.)

One gallon of petrol alone contains up to 4 grams of lead, which is discharged into the atmosphere in the vehicle's exhaust, then to be inhaled or to fall on to food to be ingested. Fortunately, its use as an antiknock additive is now declining, and lead plumbing is gradually being replaced, but we still get a hefty supplement in our food and in the air.

Food intake is less significant, as only 5 to 10 per cent of the ingested lead reaches the bloodstream (although this is 5 to 10 per cent too much). In contrast, 30 to 50 per cent of inhaled lead gets into the blood. Blood levels range from 0.05 to 0.4 ppm, and it is relatively easy for those working daily in exhaust-filled areas to reach the undesirable 0.5 ppm level.

What does lead do?
Lead accumulates in the bones, including the teeth, where it replaces calcium. Studies on human bones over 500 years old show lead levels at 5 ppm, in comparison with the more usual 50 ppm found today.

As we age, it gets stored as lead triphosphate in the liver, pancreas, kidney and major blood vessels, preventing normal maturation of our vital red blood cells and producing characteristic stippling. Normal synthesis of our blood pigment, haemoglobin, is also impaired.

Its build-up causes headaches, unusual pains, insomnia, constipation, poor concentration and irritability. Hyperactivity is common in children exposed to a lot of lead, as children are much more efficient at absorbing toxic minerals than adults.

Reducing lead
Avoid heavy traffic where possible. Include adequate fibre in the diet and take extra calcium, magnesium and vitamins C and B_1, all of which help to prevent lead uptake, or render it less harmful.

CADMIUM

We are normally born with no cadmium at all in our bodies, but we accumulate it, especially in the kidneys, liver, lungs and pancreas, as we age. When it reaches a certain level it causes tissue damage. Some people, if they smoke and are exposed to cadmium at work, e.g. in smelting plants or in the fertiliser industry, may reach this level during middle or old age, whilst others never reach it.

The effects of a build-up of cadmium were clearly shown in 1970 when inhabitants of a city in Japan (Toyana), who had for years complained of lumbago, started to develop severe bone pain. The disease was memorably named Ouch-Ouch disease and the whole skeleton became soft.

Cadmium inhibits the functions of enzymes containing the sulphydry-l (-SH-) groups and antibodies. It seems to act on the smooth muscle of blood vessels and raises blood pressure, as well as disturbing calcium metabolism. In 1942 cadmium was positively linked with some spontaneous bone fractures and cases of osteoporosis. In the 1950s it was found to interfere with the development of tooth enamel. It is known to be carcinogenic in rats, affecting the testicles in particular. It is also mutagenic, inducing malformations in the faces of newborn rats.

ALUMINIUM

Aluminium is the third most abundant element and the most abundant metal in the earth's crust, but it has never been shown to be essential to either plants or animals. Because aluminium is so reactive, it is normally found safely bound with silicon, oxygen or hydrogen in the ground. Nowadays, however, acid rain has freed a lot of this previously bound aluminium. Soluble aluminium is now available in our water and in many soils. On top of this, aluminium sulphate is sometimes added to our water supplies as a flocculant.

Most plants and animals do not absorb much aluminium, and it was thought that it was not absorbed via the human gut. This is true at low environmental levels as there is a natural gut barrier. However, our intake has increased as aluminium has become part of a variety of food additives, over-the-counter drugs such as antacids and aspirin, cooking utensils, cosmetics and water treatment. These greater concentrations have rendered our gut barrier ineffective, and aluminium is now stored in the lungs, liver, thyroid and brain. People with impaired kidney function also lay it down in the bone. Uptake varies depending on concentration, genetic susceptibility, hormone levels and nutritional status (calcium and magnesium levels being critical).

Tolerance to its presence also varies, and those with less than optimal kidney function, with diabetes, skeletal problems, immune problems or high levels of other toxic metals are obviously less tolerant. Aluminium, once absorbed, is very difficult to get rid of; it is accumulative, especially in the brain.

Toxic effects of aluminium

- Aluminium binds to DNA (the cells' genetic material).
- It is deposited in the brain, where it is the cause of abnormal neurofibrillary tangles; these have been implicated in what is probably the most well-known condition associated with high aluminium levels, Alzheimer's disease or senile dementia.
- It inhibits the enzyme hexokinase. Without this enzyme the body cannot metabolise carbohydrate effectively; it is one of the reasons why diabetics are more sensitive.
- Aluminium can cause contact dermatitis.
- It can also cause phosphate depletion and skeletal demineralisation resembling osteomalacia (softening of the bones).
- It can exacerbate osteoporosis; calcium utilisation is interfered with and so compromises bone repair and immune function.

- It has also, along with lead, been linked to slow learning and decreased visual-motor performance in children.
- Babies are at special risk from aluminium intoxication if they are on artificial feed, as their kidneys are immature; water used to make up feeds should not be high in aluminium, neither should the feed. At the time of writing, soya-based formulas were very high; it is hoped that manufacturers will have improved this by the time this book is published.
- Women at the menopause are extremely susceptible to aluminium accumulation as their hormone changes favour increased uptake of this metal.
- Excess aluminium also adversely affects haemoglobin production and interferes with iron transport.
- It is also known to be the cause of dialysis dementia.

Minimising aluminium intake

Naturally bound aluminium, even in cereals and vegetables, is not thought to be a problem to our health; it is the soluble forms, deliberately added to medicines, food or water, which cause the problems.

To avoid aluminium do not cook food, and acidic foods in particular, in aluminium pans; use stainless steel or glass for preference.

Aluminium salts are used in the food industry, mainly as emulsifying, anti-caking, bleaching and raising agents. Additives E173, 541, 554, 556, 558 and 559 should be avoided.

2I
POLLUTION OF THE AIR

Clean air, along with wholesome food and clean water, is a basic right of all living things. We cannot live without it. Today the air is not so clean, and the immune system, yet again, has to pick up the bill for our careless actions and dirty habits.

We cannot see clean air, and yet we need to take it into our lungs continuously to sustain life. On average we take in 14 to 18 breaths per minute when sitting still. If we take in clean air, the body can deal with everything, extract the oxygen it needs and leave us with clean lungs. Unfortunately these days, even if we live in a small clean town, we are liable to inhale around 40,000 specks of dust every time we breathe in; living in a dirty city we can be bombarded with 70,000 or more specks of dust with every breath.

We have simple defence mechanisms which prevent some of this dirt from entering the lungs. Nostrils produce mucus and have hairs which trap some particles. However excessive smaller-particle pollution causes over-stimulation in some sensitive people so their mucus-secreting glands either produce nasal fluids continually or give up completely. At the last count it is the immune system which has to play vacuum cleaner and get rid of the rubbish, but who empties the bag and where? We were not designed for coping with all this dirt.

When we breathe in the air goes from our nose or mouth down the trachea and into the bronchi (the air tubes) which lead into our two lungs. These both inflate (rather like a balloon does when you blow into it). Air is then taken up by the alveoli, which are the little sacs making up much of the lung tissue. If you could spread all these sacs out you would get a surface area something the size of a tennis court, all for sponging up the air that we breathe. Oxygen is then picked up by the capillaries (minute blood vessels) and goes into the bloodstream. Waste carbon dioxide comes out of the blood and is exhaled from the lungs when we breathe out.

The nose keeps out many larger dust particles, and many very small ones are breathed in and out again. It is the in-between particles that stick on to the little alveoli and clog up the works. White blood corpuscles rush out on red alert and try to clean them up, but if the exposure is daily and persistent, they are often fighting a losing battle, and disease follows.

WHAT SHOULD AIR BE?

Air is made up of roughly 77 per cent nitrogen and 21 per cent oxygen. The remaining small amount contains the inert gases, carbon dioxide and water vapour. We need the carbon dioxide to survive, although we do not use it personally; plants need it in order to make their food and we need them, both for food and to provide us with oxygen.

Indeed, almost all living things need oxygen in order to breathe, and that includes plants. Even aquatic creatures use oxygen dissolved in water. There are very few living things that do not need oxygen – some bacteria do not, and neither do cancer cells.

The nitrogen in the air is utilised by bacteria and plants so that it eventually becomes available to us, usually in the form of protein.

What else do we get?

Fire gives off all sorts of smoke, dust and undesirable gases like the nitrogen, sulphur and carbon oxides. Nature coped with these until man started using fire as a tool and progressed from wood to coal as a fuel. Way back in the 12th century people noticed that smoke made the air they breathed unpleasant, and there is a record of a man being tortured to death during the reign of Edward II for burning coal and fouling the air.

Carbon monoxide is produced at very high altitudes, but this is counterbalanced by bacteria which can convert it into carbon dioxide. At ground level certain plants, for example the common spider plant, can do the same. These are very helpful plants, and can be used to remove at least some of the contamination if you live on a busy street. Unfortunately we now make carbon monoxide quite abundantly, as it is produced as an exhaust from the internal combustion engines in cars. We do not really want it in the air we breathe; for a start, it poisons the oxygen-transporting haemoglobin in the red blood cells.

Similarly, the action of sunlight on the nitrogen dioxide in exhaust fumes produces ozone. This, again, is a gas which we need up in the stratosphere, but not down here where we have to breathe it in. It can cause thickening and deterioration of the lung tissue.

THE ATMOSPHERE

Our atmosphere is precious. It is unique to earth. It can easily be damaged, and if its chemical balance is badly disturbed it could cause the destruction of much life on earth. Its thickness averages out at something like 300 miles into space, but it is not all breathable. The bit we can breathe is a mere skin on the apple; it is called the troposphere and extends out only about 5 miles at the poles and 15 miles at the equator. Up mountains it can become very thin on oxygen so that breathing can be difficult 14,000 feet above sea level.

Above the troposphere comes the stratosphere, where we want our ozone; this ozone layer protects us from the radiation of the sun by absorbing much of the harmful radiation.

AIR POLLUTION

Before the passing of our Clean Air Act in 1956, a smog incident in London that year killed 1,000 people. In December of 1952 the smog death toll was 4,000, the worst air pollution disaster in history. Los Angeles is another area which suffers from smog problems, so in the 1950s smog alert systems were brought into effect. The first alert was a voluntary cut-down, but if the build-up of pollutants continued the second alert was a total ban on the use of cars, buses, etc., except for emergencies.

We are all agreed that nobody wants air pollution, and nobody likes it. The trouble is, we all like the things that make it.

Cars, boats and planes

Our cars are one of the major contributors to air pollution. A million cars using leaded petrol cough up 2,000 tons of lead per year; they also release around 660,000 tons of carbon monoxide, 60,000 tons of nitrogen oxides and 10,000 tons of sulphur oxides. Just think how many millions of cars there must be in the world.

Traffic jams are even worse sources of pollution. They often occur in built-up areas where people are walking close to the exhaust pipes; children are particularly vulnerable as toddlers and push-chairs are much nearer exhaust-pipe levels. A car speeding along emits around 10 micrograms of the carcinogenic benzopyrene a minute, but when it is stuck in a traffic jam it throws out 234 micrograms of benzopyrene per minute. If anyone suggested that our babies and toddlers should inhale this as a daily supplement, doctors, health professionals and probably even politicians would throw up their hands in horror at the suggestion, arguing that not only was there no benefit to the supplement, but there are also many potential hazards. Yet this is effectively what is happening.

We have had internal combustion engines for a very short period of time in man's history, but have become dependent on them for our accepted lifestyles, and now almost everyone in the western world uses buses or cars frequently. Many of us have changed to lead-free so-called 'clean' cars in an attempt to keep lead out of our air, but even these still produce nitric oxides and other air pollutants. We may one day have to choose between our cars or our air, and find that we cannot do without either.

Another staggering statistic is that a four-engine jet taking off from one of our airports uses the equivalent amount of fuel to 8,000 cars each driving for one hour. These hungry metal birds spew out a corresponding large amount of exhaust (and noise pollution). Supersonic aircraft may also damage the ozone layer in our stratosphere.

Industry
Industry is another major source of air pollution, belching out tons of sulphur, lead, zinc, carbon and nitrogen oxides, fluorides, hydrogen sulphide, chlorine and ammonia into our air and hence into our lungs. Ironically food processing plants are one of the major offenders, along with those that make chemicals, paper, steel, aluminium and rubber. In a few cases, high hydrogen fluoride and sulphur emissions have caused people in the surrounding area to be ill, to develop asthma and other breathing problems, as well as skin, heart and emotional problems. Smokestacks are being built higher so that pollutants are distributed over a greater area (giving more people a chance to sample a little bit); the more expensive, but healthier, option would be to clean or neutralise the emissions first.

How does air pollution affect our health?
We know that excessive inhalation of silicon dust causes silicosis and asthma; that taking in asbestos causes asbestosis and lung cancer; that many coalminers suffer with pneumoconiosis (black lung disease); that textile workers working in an enclosed environment can contract byssinosis (brown lung disease).

We know that breathing in lead particles can affect the nervous system and brain; that carbon monoxide combines with the pigment in our blood and so prevents normal uptake of oxygen, really high levels causing blood clots or even heart failure. Ozone weakens the immune system and makes the body less resistant to bugs; it also causes a thickening and blocking of lung tissue and encourages depression.

We know that prolonged exposure to sulphur dioxide is linked to heart attacks, cancer and genetic changes and that the action of water on this sulphur dioxide turns it into sulphuric acid which damages the lungs. People with high exposure to this become much more prone to respiratory diseases.

Research is showing that people who are continually exposed to plane exhausts have a greater risk of developing dementia – illnesses such as Parkinson's or Alzheimer's disease.

Beryllium causes inflammation of the eye, skin and lung tissue, and smoking can cause coughing, bronchitis, cancer and heart disease. Someone who smokes one packet of cigarettes per day takes in about 60 micrograms of the carcinogenic hydrocarbon benzo-pyrene, on top of other air pollution. This is regarded as bad, but before our Clean Air Act in London even a non-smoker could have been getting 320 micrograms of benzopyrene a day, which is equivalent to five packets of cigarettes. Fortunately, London's air is no longer this bad, but there is no reason to slacken our efforts at cleaning up the air. The benzopyrene is of course not the only damaging factor in cigarettes.

Herbicides can be breathed in if spread by plane, causing breathing problems and even genetic mutations.

Pollution in the home

Not all of our air pollution is outdoors; we can create our own heavily polluted environment in our homes.

Fires and smoking are sources of indoor air pollution. Gas from cookers or central heating is another, and a few people can be sensitive to this; it can make them very ill, with headaches, depression, and sometimes asthma or joint pains, the symptoms disappearing completely if they go on holiday in all-electric accommodation. Gas is lighter than air and so tends to go all over the house if it escapes. Oil and paraffin heaters can also cause allergy and other health problems.

At home or at work we breathe in such things as floor polishes, detergents, disinfectants, aerosols, fly sprays, furniture polish, perfumes, deodorants, bacterial spores from biological washing powders, paint and air fresheners. At work, air conditioning may have the additional function of adding pollutants.

We tend to ignore such air pollution, especially at home, because we usually cannot see it. Furthermore, these days many people are zinc deficient, which lessens their sense of smell so they do not smell the air pollution either. But it is there, and it has an effect on our health.

Perhaps air pollution is a contributory factor in causing the sleeplessness and depression which makes millions of people these days turn to sleeping pills, tranquillisers and anti-depressants.

CONCLUSION

We need to be aware of our air pollutants and do our best to keep the levels down. After all, breathing is pretty essential to life. Apart from the adverse effects it has on our own immune systems and health, it would be dreadful to think of our children's children, walking or cycling from place to place wearing their own mini atmosphere and pulling in at air stations for refills, all because of us. Science fiction it may be, but perhaps we will be forced to go forward into the past.

We are still children on this planet and need to be careful about trying to run before we can walk. I once read that if we put the history of earth into a timescale that we could comprehend, and took one year as the timescale from earth as a gaseous ball to the present day, then it would only have been a month ago that plant life developed and man as a species would only have lived three and a half hours. Jesus would have been born in the last 12 seconds and Columbus would have discovered America in the last three seconds. Now try to visualise that one year as the estimated five billion years that earth has been in existence. Man is very new – the dinosaur was around for much longer than we have been on the earth's surface. If we do not wish to become extinct too, we need to take a less selfish view of the world. We need to stop acting without first considering if our actions will damage anything and if we can clean up afterwards. What is the point of negotiating a higher salary and a better standard of living if our children cannot live to enjoy it?

Hindsight is a wonderful thing. No one started out with the intention of poisoning our environment but now that we can see the effects, it is time to alter our ways. We can all do our little bit of cleaning up. No one is immune from the effects of pollution of our food, land, water and air. They are the things we all share.

22
MAKING A MOVE

EXERCISE

The immune system needs exercise, muscular contraction, in order to move lymph around the body. The lymphatic system does not have a pump, like the heart, which is used to pump blood around, but relies on muscular contraction to push the lymph through the lymph nodes and along the lymphatic vessels. In one experiment with rats, carbon particles were found to travel from the thigh to the chest of a rat in 20 minutes when there was muscular activity; however, when the rat was rested for 24 hours, there was no evidence of lymphatic transport at all. Lymph is heavier when it contains a lot of fat, so a high fat diet and not much exercise is a recipe for a stagnant, inefficient lymph and hence a sluggish immune system.

Cars are a relatively new invention. There are many people alive today who remember travelling by horse, or horse and carriage, because there were very few cars in their youth. Our bodies are designed to be active and they have not as yet adapted to the new sedentary lifestyle. They may not even do so, though I do vividly remember reading a science fiction book in which humans rolled round like wobbly men because our bodies had evolved to the point where they did not form legs as they were no longer necessary.

Today, though, humans need action or they lose their strength, bone tissue, flexibility, muscle tone, agility, elasticity, lung capacity, heart tone, immune function, energy, and probably a whole lot of other things. They need daily, slow, gentle stretching and bending movements of the body, as well as exercises like walking which maintain the calcium content of the bones.

It is known that exercise alters the fat profile of the blood for the better. It also strengthens the heart, decreases the resting pulse rate and increases a sense of well-being by causing the production of hormone-like chemicals called endorphins. Vigorous exercise also disperses corticosteroids produced during stress; if not dispersed, these corticosteroids cause the thymus and lymph nodes to shrink, and interferon and T-cell production to decrease.

Exercise also improves circulation, thus increasing both oxygen supply to tissues and toxic waste removal. Lung capacity is one of the first characteristics to decrease with age, but exercise helps to maintain this capacity, especially exercises which control breathing or call for holding the breath. Swimming, though good for the heart and the lungs, does not help to retain bone density. So swimming is not good as the only form of exercise if you are past middle age, as it does not help in preventing osteoporosis.

Top athletes do not necessarily live longer than the rest of us, neither are they exempt from heart disease, so exercise is only part of the story. Indeed top athletes often over-train; to reach the peak of their career, they may go over the top of their peak for health. Do not over-exercise; always warm up muscles first, especially if they are not used to being used, and make sure you get enough nutrients to cope with the activity.

Exercise need not be difficult; you do not have to be able to participate in some sport or pay to go to complex leisure centres in order to get the exercise that you need to stay healthy. Walking is excellent; so are bending and stretching exercises, perhaps to music if that is what you prefer. The main aim is to contract and relax all the muscles you can find at least once a week, and the most obvious ones every day. There are lots of books on exercises, so it is not my intention to go into these here. The important thing is to enjoy the exercise which you choose, and to build up slowly if you are not used to it.

Advantages of movement
Depending on age, weight, etc., movement which increases the heart beat sufficiently for around 20 minutes per day would be extremely valuable in:

- Either maintaining normal or reducing high blood pressure.
- Either maintaining a low or reducing a high resting pulse rate.
- Changing the fat profile of the blood in favour of less harmful fats.
- Maintaining normal body weight and muscle tone.
- Increasing the sense of well-being and improving self-image.
- Keeping the immune army on the move; remember it is muscular contraction which keeps the lymph moving and allows transport of immune soldiers.
- Increasing energy levels.
- Dispersing toxins which build up in a sedentary body.
- Strengthening bones (minerals come out of bones whilst sleeping or if we have a sedentary lifestyle). Exercise helps to deposit minerals in the bone bank.

BREATHING

Breathing is a forgotten exercise, but very important. These days we all shallow-breathe, and rarely do anything else. This hastens the degeneration of the lungs. Exercise which regularly calls for deep breathing is therefore important. If you are not into running, etc., then deep breaths or singing will do very nicely – people who sing a lot retain lung elasticity.

Breathing, as well as lifting and stretching exercises, are especially important for the disabled or elderly. Not only does it keep their muscles, bones, heart and lungs happy, but it also improves immune function. Small babies move little; they do not know how to, and it is at this time that whooping cough can be a killer – death is caused by lung collapse, because the lungs are not strong enough. Later, a weak sickly child is more prone to infection than one who runs around exercising and strengthening their lungs and immune function.

RELAXATION

Relaxation is as important as movement, but oddly enough, although many people lead sedentary lives, they often find it difficult to relax. They slump into ill-fitting chairs, strain the spine, cause constriction of the blood flow by crossing their legs or lying on an arm; they crunch up the body organs, especially the stomach and intestines, often whilst nibbling or after having eaten a meal. Then they wonder why they have indigestion, which increases the pain and stress and calls for an antacid. This puts an end to digestion completely, and only feeds the bugs in the intestines, leaving incompletely digested food which causes gas and constipation. Call this relaxation?

SLEEP

Sleep is still a mystery, but it is a major factor in health problems. On average, we all spend a total of about 20 years of our life sleeping. It is essential for life – after less than 20 days deprived of sleep, death occurs.

It seems that in real sleep we produce a sleep-inducing substance which brings about sleep and is present in the blood. Experiments on rabbits showed that the blood from sleeping rabbits, when injected into awake rabbits, caused them to go to sleep. The substance which was thought to induce sleep was made up of nine different amino acids.

During sleep the blood pressure drops by anything from 10 to 30 points, although a really exciting dream may raise it a lot; this is sometimes a problem for heart patients, who wake in the early hours with a racing pulse and high blood pressure. Pulse rate normally drops by about 20 beats per minute during sleep and temperature and metabolic rate also fall.

Production of fluids like urine, tears and saliva fall, sometimes causing dry eyes and sore throat on waking. Sweat production, however, increases and sweat takes with it a lot of toxins that we have accumulated during the day.

Delta sleep, which takes place during stages three and four of human sleep, is very important for the immune function as it is during this stage that the pituitary gland steps up production of growth hormone, which in turn stimulates the thymus gland.

REM sleep
REM sleep – sleep characterised by rapid eye movements and recollection of dreams after being awakened from them – is also essential for health. REM sleep is linked with speech, memory storage and learning; when deprived of it, learning becomes more difficult. Telling children, or indeed adults, stories before bed not only relaxes them, but encourages lengthy REM sleep and so probably improves learning ability. Exercise, though not immediately before bed, also improves sleep by increasing deeper levels of non-REM sleep. Noises in sleep do alter dream patterns, although they do not necessarily awaken us; we need dark and quiet for healthy undisturbed sleep. Even alcohol suppresses REM sleep, and its continued use, or the continued use of barbiturates, tranquillisers and amphetamines, alter the rhythm of REM sleep and it is difficult to get back to a normal pattern.

Work on patients that have had a stroke or serious accident depriving them of speech has shown that they are also deficient in REM sleep. If speech returned, then so did normal REM sleep; if it was not restored, neither was REM sleep. Interestingly, Helen Keller, who was blind and deaf from birth, could only communicate using smell, taste and touch. Eventually she taught herself to speak, and only then could she see in her dreams and describe what she saw.

Dreaming
Many people think that they do not dream, but what they really mean is that they do not recall them. This may be due to a vitamin B, in

particular B$_6$, deficiency. Alternatively they may remember dreams only for an instant after waking, or have a longer period after REM sleep before waking properly.

Some cultures believe that real life is only for acting out important parts of dreams, and that it is our dream life which is real and significant. Bertrand Russell used this theme when he portrayed real life as a persistent nightmare in his book *Human Knowledge*. Certainly, daydreaming can be one of life's greatest pleasures, and a great way to relax if you allow yourself to enjoy the fantasy, but it can be unpleasant and stress inducing if you dwell on problems or thoughts of fear and pain.

Insomnia
We all need different amounts of sleep, depending on age, activity, metabolism, diet, condition and life circumstances. The amount of sleep needed will change; a lot of insomnia is caused by worrying about insomnia which does not exist. We all have periods in life when more or less sleep is needed.

Famous insomniacs are Louis XIV of France, who had 413 beds so that he could always find the right one for the best sleep, and Benjamin Franklin, who had a modest four in his bedroom but whose wife complained that she could never find him in the dark. Other insomniacs take a more light-hearted view; Mark Twain said 'If you can't sleep, try lying on the end of the bed and you might drop off'. Napoleon would only sleep if his feet pointed north.

L-tryptophan is used as a dietary aid for alleviating insomnia, although the stages of sleep and the sleep cycle do not appear to be altered by its supplementation. It increases serotonin levels, which are sleep inducing, and sometimes it also brings about the return of normal REM sleep if this has been lost.

A single night's sleeping pill is probably no worse at disturbing the rhythm than a long trans-Atlantic flight; such sleeping pills on odd occasions are relatively harmless; but many drugs used to induce sleep give an artificial state with side effects. Some only cause drowsiness, and more often do not bring about sleep. Many are addictive and cause nightmares, especially on withdrawal of the drug; it is ironic that one often has to endure sleepless nights and extreme anxiety in order to get off drugs which were taken in the first place to cure the problem of insomnia. Many such drugs also produce dreamless sleep and seriously interfere with REM sleep.

CONCLUSION

Exercise, relaxation and sleep are essential for good health and an efficient immune system. We need a good balance, with not too much or too little of any of them. The pattern of need will change often in life and becomes obvious if you get to know yourself and become aware of your own body language.

There are times, at work for example, where you cannot go to sleep or go for a run, although your body might tell you that it would like to. But in between these times there has to be a time for you, when you can listen to your body's requirements. If there isn't, then you are too busy and are living in overdrive.

23
THE SOUND OF SILENCE

Silence is indeed golden, but noise makes gold. Our cars and planes, boats and trains, mowers and washing machines, saws and hoovers, all make noise. Places of entertainment and recreation also make noise, as well as money.

Noise is any sort of sound, but we usually use the word noise to describe a sound that we find disturbing or unpleasant. However, what one person may call noise, another may call music; some sounds are pleasant to some people and not to others. Some noises we become accustomed to and do not take any outward notice of them; people who live in the country find the city noisy, whilst city dwellers have become accustomed to it. Although we outwardly switch off to noise, our subconscious is always switched on to it and it can have a dramatic effect on the immune system. We need sound because we use it for communication and we can use it for relaxation and pleasure, but silence is also of the utmost importance in maintaining good health.

NOISE AND ILLNESS

We no longer spend hours reading books; instead we use television, radio, recordplayers, tapes, etc. Such very loud sounds for long stretches can be very damaging, and not only to our hearing. After a while the whole body, and in particular the blood system, becomes involved, making the individual very tired.

A loud bang can disintegrate many of the hair cells that detect sound in our cochlea (inner ear) and they will not be replaced. It can also cause constriction of the tiny blood vessels in the whole body and may deprive the inner ear of blood, causing further destruction of many of our hearing cells. And unfortunately noise damage is cumulative. Because it often does not cause pain we do not tend to avoid it, but the sad truth is that once hearing has gone for this reason, it has gone for ever.

At the other end of the scale, infrasound (very low noises) has been found to cause intense pain in the stomach, heart and lungs, and has been researched for use as a weapon of war or for riot control. We cannot hear infrasound; it vibrates at less than 15 cycles per second and we can only feel it.

Noises will have different effects on other animals. Dogs and horses, for example, hear sounds over 20,000 cycles per second (above the range of human hearing), and bats use these higher sounds to navigate; dolphins may even use them to communicate with one another. Ultrasound can be employed to kill insects or to get rid of bugs in milk. Our noise pollution may therefore be having dramatic effects on other animals.

NOISE AND SLEEP

We are particularly vulnerable to noise when we are asleep. The quality of sleep has been shown (by measuring brain waves) to be disturbed, even if the sleeper has not been suffering from insomnia and was not aware of the impaired sleep patterns. This link between noise pollution, sleep problems and general well-being is not new; Julius Caesar, back in the first century BC, banned chariots from the cobbled streets at night because of the disturbance the noise caused.

Noise could be contributing to our national ills. Sudden noises causes rapid heart beat, raised blood pressure and contraction of blood vessels. Over a period of time, with continual noise stimulation, these conditions could possibly become the norm. Rabbits and rats exposed to our noise have developed clogged blood vessels and had heart attacks and strokes. Noise may thus be a contributory factor in heart and circulatory diseases, as well as in immune related diseases. It also causes a tightening of the whole digestive tract and reduces the flow of saliva and gastric juices aggravating digestive problems.

Thyroid hormone production is affected by noise and this can cause emotional problems. A particularly disturbing study on rats showed that noise had a direct effect on the thymus gland, which is, of course, the master gland of the immune system. Noise also causes the adrenal glands to be over-stimulated and interferes with kidney function; it exacerbates allergy problems, including bedwetting and mental illness.

NOISE DAMAGE

The Mabaan people live in the African Sudan. They live peacefully and simply; the normal sound level in a Mabaan village is below 40 decibels. It has been found that the average 75-year-old Mabaan has hearing comparable to the average 25-year-old in this country. Deafness does not automatically come with old age: we hasten it with too much noise.

Noise is potentially damaging to all things. It makes the very air vibrate and can cause glass to shatter. So how much more sensitive are living things to its force. Exposure to noise of more than 85 decibels for any prolonged period of time can damage our delicate hearing mechanism. When the noise reaches 120 decibels you can actually feel it and over 140 decibels it hurts. Non-living things can become damaged at 155 decibels and over, depending on the material.

Anything which disturbs sleep obviously increases fatigue. Two thousand years ago the Chinese used continual noise as a torture, its effect being insanity followed by death. Women are much more likely to be disturbed by noise during sleep than men.

NOISE AND EMOTIONS

All noise and no stillness makes for over-stimulation, which eventually drains both our mental and physical energy. Schools now are introducing USSR, which stands for uninterrupted sustained silent reading; it means that pupils have a reading book which is within their capabilities and they have to read silently for half an hour or so without help or interruption. It is a good idea to encourage everyone to have a period of silence during each day, to give them a rest from the constant stimulation of noise which encourages hyperactivity and jittery behaviour.

Emotionally, noise can create anxiety, tension, irritation, apprehension and even great fear; research suggests that it can make some people more aggressive and prone to quarrels and anger. It is interesting to note that it is not always just the noise itself that is destructive, but also our attitude to it, because this affects our emotions as well.

Silence is very important. We need it for maximum concentration. We need it for sorting out our own thoughts and feelings. We need it for mental healing and inner peace. We need it to relax the grip of tension on our muscles and blood vessels, and to slow our body chemistry, including the immune system, to a healthier, more manageable pace.

Silence is essential to our well-being and we may not be getting enough of it. Try to treat yourself to a little every day and feel the benefit. It is cheap, but often difficult to find.

24
LET THERE BE LIGHT

Man was designed to work in natural light, and he was intended to have periods of light and darkness. Research is now beginning to show links between our exposure to natural light, or the lack of it, and its effect on our immune system and general health. Just as it is possible to become ill because of sounds which we cannot hear but which affect the body, especially the gut (cf previous chapter on noise), so it is possible to be affected by light.

Some exposure to the ultraviolet in daylight promotes health and healing; everyone knows that they feel better in the summer or during winter holidays abroad when they can go outside. These days we tend to live behind glass, especially in the winter, using artificial lights, television and computer screens, etc. Some research has linked this as a contributory factor to the increase in hyperactivity and behavioural or learning problems in children, as well as depression, tiredness and lack of concentration in people in general. One group of researchers filmed a group of schoolchildren under artificial light and under natural light; they found the group to be much calmer and less fidgety in natural light.

Natural light is especially important for children, as it stimulates growth hormone and lessens the severity of childhood illnesses by stimulating the immune system via the thymus. It is also important, as we get older, to maintain the activity of the thymus and hence the immune system.

It seems that light in the blue range can promote healing, and may even help to reduce blood pressure. Blue light promotes peace and relaxation. It is sometimes of benefit to those who suffer from headaches.

Red, on the other hand, stimulates. Whilst lighting of this colour can be used to increase activity in offices and other places of work, it is not good for people with a tendency to cancer to be exposed to red light too often. Several studies on mice show that they develop tumours very quickly when forced to live under pink illumination; these mice, as would be expected, had the shortest life. Mice who lived in natural light lived longest and those living under glass but in normal dark/daylight conditions came next. It is a long way from mouse to man, but why use pink or red light when it could be a contributory factor to the development of cancer and a shortened life-span? We were, after all, adapted to live in natural light. The sea, the sky, the plants, the things which we would naturally look at for most of the day, are blues and greens. We only get periodic flashes of red in flowers, sunrises and sunsets. Could there be a reason? Can we be over-stimulated?

Natural light is free and of great benefit to the immune system and health. It has no nasty side effects (unless we destroy the ozone layer or allow ourselves to be burnt). So a daily supplement of natural light is definitely worth trying.

Darkness is also free and necessary, so do not be tempted to sleep regularly with the light on. If you are the sort of person who does, arrange a time switch to turn it off and an easy way to turn the light on should you awake in the dark.

LIGHT AND DISEASE

Natural and artificial light affect all living things.
- Plants respond to light, bending their shoots towards it, whilst the roots grow away from it.
- Length of day is known to affect bird migration.
- Shorter winter days decrease chicken egg production, so artificial light is used to lengthen the day and keep egg production up.
- Artificial blue light is used in hospitals, in particular for pre-term babies who show signs of jaundice.
- The endocrine system, which makes our hormones, responds to visible light.
- Ultraviolet or black light is used to treat psoriasis and acne.

It is even possible that the change in light, as well as in nutrients, affects viruses or our immune response to them. Work on the tomato virus showed it to be more common in cloudy weather or at times of low light intensity. In one experiment, where diseased tomatoes were exposed to natural light instead of light filtered through their greenhouse glass, they reverted to healthy plants. Perhaps our winter virus epidemics could be lessened if we were not indoors so much.

Like plants, we need nutrients and light to work at our best. Light therapy is not an extensively researched area, but there is a very logical thread running through the theory. We know that, in general, we live behind glass and that air pollution has cut our natural light supply to such an extent that in some heavily polluted areas certain crops will no longer grow there. So it is worth trying to get a bit more light into our daily lives. It is still readily available, though not as easily as in the days of windows that opened!

Arthritis

Natural light may be of great importance if you have a tendency to suffer from arthritis. One American consultant had to retire from surgery because his arthritis had become so bad. He spent his days in the garden and his arthritis improved to such an extent that he took up medicine again and started helping others with this condition. He also helped to develop a glass which allows more natural light to pass through, and a light bulb which delivers light much closer to the natural light spectrum than the artificial lights that we normally use.

Although still a little-tried therapy, it is worth being your own guinea-pig if you suffer from this condition. At worst you may experience no relief, but you will have lost nothing. At best, there could be a great improvement in mobility and a lessening of pain.

Seasonal affective disorder

Half a million British people are estimated to suffer from seasonal affective disorder (SAD), in which their bodies suffer from natural light deficiency due to the decrease in daylight and a tendency to stay indoors. SAD people are depressed during the winter, eat more and sleep more. The pineal gland produces more melatonin in the dark, and this induces sleep. It also seems to stimulate the desire for alcohol. When subjected to extended darkness, even rats choose to drink alcohol in preference to water, if they are given the choice.

It should be noted that ordinary strip lighting is not a good way to rectify this situation, as there is some concern that this type of lighting causes depression in itself. There is nothing quite like daylight.

Skin cancer

The one well-publicised side effect of sunlight is skin cancer. But as with so much else, balance is the key.

Too much or too little of anything can kill. We need oxygen, for example, to live, yet if we have too much of it, it will kill us; if the oxygen content of the air went up a mere 2 per cent, from 23 to 25 per cent, we would probably suffer from lung disease. On top of that, the environmental effects would be devastating, with melting ice caps and spontaneous fires. Similarly, we need a good amount of natural light and a balancing amount of darkness. We do not need our artificial light for health, but it is very convenient and we would not want to do without it; however, to maintain good health, we need to achieve a good working balance.

It is also important to know which type of person you are. An arthritic sufferer who has worn glasses most of his life is likely to be light deficient, and needs to increase exposure to daylight, without glasses on. An outdoor fisherman or farmer, who does not wear glasses at all, does not need any more. An office worker would probably be better off not wearing sunglasses outdoors during his luncheon break. Constant wearing of sunglasses that filter out the ultraviolet light actually increases the need for the glasses; the pupil stays wider open than it would do if ultraviolet light was allowed through and so the rest of the visible light seems brighter. Natural light falling on the eyes is beneficial to the immune system as it stimulates the thymus.

Sudden prolonged exposure to sunlight is not, however, the best way to get your sunlight. If you think about it, an office worker who avoids exposure to sunlight throughout the year, but goes on holiday for two weeks and lies in strong sunshine every day, all day, is bound to have problems. It is like someone who rarely drinks alcohol getting drunk every day for two weeks. Sunlight is more likely to be damaging from about 11 am to 2 pm, when there are greater amounts of the more harmful UVB. So, if on holiday, especially abroad, organise lunch in the shade or some other indoor-shaded activity during this period. However if you are working in Britain and making the best of an hour's lunch break, the timing is unlikely to be a problem. The key is, again, a good balance; a gradual build-up and a tailing-off of exposure to sunlight throughout the seasons.

It is never a good idea to get sunburnt and to damage the skin. Neither is it a good idea to avoid it completely. Sunbeds are rarely advisable, as it is difficult to know if they have the right ultraviolet balance.

The second way to prevent skin cancer is to ensure one has adequate natural protection. Some drugs and also nutrient deficiencies cause a few people to become very sensitive to natural light. Phenylalanine, an ingredient of many soft diet drinks, is food for a melanoma (skin cancer), so go easy on the intake of these drinks when on holiday. Beta-carotene is a great natural skin protector. A combination of para-amino benzoic acid (PABA), pantothenic acid and folic acid allows you to maximise your own melanin production and so increase natural protection; deficiencies in these B vitamins and in vitamin B$_2$ will cause sensitivity to light and squinting. It is not a bad idea to maximise this protection a week before going on holiday and during it by taking 15,000 iu in beta-carotene, 500 mg PABA, 250 mg pantothenic acid and a 50 mg B complex every other day, taking the supplements in the morning, preferably without alcohol. This will increase your ability to tan and offer some protection as well (children need only half of this every third day). It will not stop you burning, though, so be sensible with exposure.

These supplements may have the added benefit of restoring colour to prematurely greying hair if it was the lack of production of pigment which caused the greying in the first place.

Another important factor in the prevention of skin cancer is our biochemical balance. Too much sodium or salt in the body (see Chapter 10) may well be one of the contributory factors that makes the skin so sensitive to ultra-violet light.

Sunlight should not be totally avoided for fear of skin cancer, but you need to be sensible about the time and duration of exposure. Natural light is not only beneficial; it is essential for good health.

25
MIND OVER IMMUNITY

Just as we are what we eat, drink and breathe, we are also what we do and what we think. Our minds and personalities are built up from, and made out of, the thoughts with which they are fed. We need to consider our thought intake and the ability of our minds to make us ill, to help us heal or to keep us fit. Harnessing the power of our thoughts, we can lift our immune systems from a courageous struggling army, forever battling against disease, into a triumphant stable army fighting for the joys of life.

We tend to divide the body into bits, and we have specialists who understand the workings of each part; there is so much to know that one individual could not possibly know all of it in depth. However, a surgeon's skill is only part of a cure for some diseases. The body has to heal the wound and heal itself. In order to do that we need a more general, holistic approach. The ancient Chinese and Greeks, Socrates in particular, knew that you could not completely heal the body without the help of the mind. Hopefully, future medicine will go forward into the past, taking with it our invaluable modern medical knowledge but not discounting or neglecting our equally precious inheritance.

Man is not just the sum of all the bits of which he is made. He has a personal control over all those bits, if he knows how to use it.

THOUGHT AND THE IMMUNE SYSTEM

It has been shown that we can increase the size of the thymus, and even the number of T lymphocytes, by the way we think. Similarly, under prolonged unpleasant stress, the thymus and lymph nodes shrink. People who cultivate unhealthy negative thoughts and life-styles become more prone to illness because this type of thinking and living can be just as devastating to the body as environmental pollution and food additives, although fortunately they are to a larger extent under our own control. We can change them.

The skin, hair and eyes react visibly to our emotions and feelings.

Even those that are endowed with apparently flawless skin and thick hair will have noticed that when they are sick and feel awful, it is the hair, eyes and skin that lack lustre first. When a person is in love or on top of the world, skin, hair and eyes visibly improve. Teenagers know that approaching exams, lack of confidence and/or other distressing emotions bring out the biggest and reddest of spots. Unhappiness and helplessness are reflected in the eyes. We also have a T cell-mediated skin response which may well reflect how the other T cells in the rest of the immune system are performing.

Several researchers and therapists have used visualisation techniques successfully. The patient visualises, for example, his immune army, swords drawn, galloping up to a cancer cell and successfully destroying it. Other people may prefer the immune army to be space invaders, zapping the cancer cells with phaser guns. Others vacuum their cancer cells away. It all depends on the individual and how he can make this therapy work for him.

Research has also shown how the brain and immune system interact via receptors and chemicals. The study of psycho-immunology and psycho-neuro-immunology is new in name at least, but may well play a large part in preventing illness and promoting healing in years to come. The good news is that it is possible to teach your immune system to become more efficient. Macrophages, for example, are less effective and less mobile when we are depressed. Chemicals which suppress the immune system are released when we are unhappy.

The most important mind factors for boosting health and the immune system are:

- To have enough positive feelings and emotions to balance out all those negative ones.
- To take a positive attitude when dealing with life's problems. It is not the problems themselves that cause damage but the way we react to them.

It does not do to dwell for too long on the unhappy and depressing thoughts, especially if we cannot change them. We need to learn whatever lessons we can from less pleasant experiences, adapt our lifestyles accordingly and get on with living. To brood continually over problems and anxieties will only cause dis-ease and hence a weakened immune system and all the symptoms of disease.

THOUGHTS, FEELINGS, EMOTIONS AND ATTITUDES

Life is not always fair. It is not always painless and trouble free;

indeed, we need life's problems in order to learn, for our personality to grow and for us to appreciate the good things in life. Often, people do not appreciate love, friendship, happiness, health, integrity, peace of mind, mobility, etc., until they have lost them. People who have nearly lost their lives often live much fuller and richer lives afterwards, realising that life is for living not for wasting or existing from day to day.

There are many feelings that will dampen our spirits and suppress the immune system if we dwell on them for too long. Sadness and bereavement are the most obvious. It is necessary to grieve. Crying is a great help for everyone as it not only relieves tension, but also washes away toxic chemicals produced by our distress. On analysis, it has been found that tears caused by peeling onions are little more than salt water compared to the complex chemical cocktail produced when tears are the result of distress. But it is not a good idea to sit on the sad fence for too long; we need to gather together the happy memories, learn the lessons that we were offered by the experience and move on to more positive thoughts.

Cancer can be a terrible illness, not only because of the disease itself, but because of the emotional cloud that it casts over the lives of its victims and their families. Is this a death sentence? Will it come back? Will it spread? These are all questions not far from the surface. Yet many people have used their cancer, or heart disease or other illness, to get more out of life. Elizabeth Rivers wrote 'I am learning more and more deeply what a precious gift this cancer has been, teaching me how to live.' Her attitude and that of many others has turned a problem into an asset; indeed, illness, disability and pain, mental or physical, has often motivated great deeds or works and created great personalities. In some cases, the body may not always work as we would like it to, but it is still possible to live a beautiful life in the mind. It is our attitude to life's problems that determines what we get out of life.

Loneliness is a great immune suppressor, and it is not just confined to people who live alone. It is possible to feel lonely when surrounded by people. School or parties can be very lonely places if you do not fit in. Many married people are lonely even when their partner is with them, because they do not feel that they belong. If that deep need to be needed or loved, or even just considered, is not satisfied, loneliness could be the result.

Similarly, dissatisfaction with life, low self-esteem, or feeling trapped in situations that are not of your own choosing, also reduces immune power, as do feelings of envy, aggression, hate, hostility, revenge, anger and guilt. Forgiveness is not easy in practice. It is easy to know that you should forgive. It is quite another thing actually to forgive – and often the most difficult person to forgive is yourself, even though not forgiving yourself can cause the most distress. If you live with the continual thought that everything is your fault and you cannot do anything right, then you are constantly criticising rather than encouraging yourself and it can have a definite detrimental effect on health. We need to be able to forgive ourselves as well as others. We will all have negative thoughts some time during our lives. It is not wrong, we are not alone, but we can change them.

Staleness, lack of interest or enthusiasm for anything and boredom are also immune suppressors. The mind needs to be creative, to think for itself, to have variety, interest and balance in its thoughts. Our minds are not machines, nor are they just lumps of meat. They get upset if we do not use them, if we constantly feed them habitual or junk thoughts. It is medicine to the mind when we feed in the 'thought vitamins' of interest and enthusiasm. Assuming there is no brain damage, Alzheimer's disease or something similar, the mind can give back whatever you want or need during life. However, it can only give back what you have put in in the first place, so it is worth filling a lot of beautiful memories, useful thoughts, imagination and dreams – they are all helpful tools in achieving a balanced mind. Do not feel guilty about spending a few minutes daydreaming, think of it as mental exercise!

Have you noticed that a lot of feelings are catching? If someone laughs, people around often smile or start laughing too – even before they know the joke. If you enter a workplace feeling really crabby, people tend to avoid you or become defensive or crabby too. Alternatively, you can walk into a room where everyone else is already hostile and soon wish that you had never entered the place. Sometimes, if your feelings are really strong and positive, you can change a whole roomful of crabs into smiling almost-human people.

Very often people, including ourselves, will be exactly what we expect them to be. If you expect someone to be lazy and uncooperative, they somehow sense it and continue to be that way. If we go into a project lacking enthusiasm and confidence, we stand a much greater chance of failing. If we accept disease with the 'It'll be the death of me' attitude, it probably will. Our attitudes to life's treasures and problems are vital keys to immune power. If we can think positive, plan our thoughts and give some time and consideration to reorganising our feelings, we would gain not only immune power but also more happiness and confidence.

Our thoughts, feelings and emotions are in our power. If we do not like some of them, we can change them. A hardening of attitudes can, I am sure, be as destructive as a hardening of the arteries, the difference being that the former are reversible, if we make the effort. It is true that it's just as difficult to change thought patterns as to alter diet, and it is always easy to drift into habitual ways. The mental diet will be constantly changing, depending on the prizes or blows one is dealt during life, but thought can be changed to encourage a less hostile environment and to boost immune power.

There is no doubt that the best atmosphere in which to work and live is the one in which everyone is happy and friendly towards each other, allowing one another the space to do their own thing, but offering help when it is needed. Such an atmosphere has to be created and worked at.

THOUGHT VITAMINS

Below are a few useful 'thought vitamins' that may help in achieving a more positive attitude to life. They can be taken when necessary. Add to your own collection of thought remedies and swap with other people.

- Laugh at least once a day. It is good for the digestion as well as your emotional well being.
- Enthusiasm gives you energy and radiance.
- Boredom makes you boring and tired.
- If you decide to do something, do it wholeheartedly not half-heartedly.
- Feelings are infectious. Friendly feelings are healthier.
- Posture conveys your attitude to others. Feel tall, walk tall. Slouch, and everyone knows that you cannot be bothered.
- A gem of humour is very precious. Smile at others' jokes. You feel better, they feel better and it does not cost you anything.
- Happiness and confidence causes secretions of endorphins in the body which further increase our feelings of well-being, and boost the immune system.
- A body thrives if its mind is trained in beautiful thoughts. Paint such thought pictures on the walls of your mind.
- We all make mistakes – all of us.
- 'When you do something good, no one remembers. When you do something wrong, no one ever forgets.' This is the wrong way around!

- Think 'build-you-up thoughts' whilst washing up or doing any other routine chores.
- Hard work is good for you as long as you enjoy it.
- It is important to recognise your own weaknesses. We all have them, but we should not let them cause further weakening.
- Sadness is necessary sometimes, but should not be dwelt on for too long.
- Blows in life will sometimes knock you down. That is no reason to crawl for the rest of your life. Get back up and go in another direction, or just try again.
- An accumulation of small difficulties can sometimes sap more of your energy than one big problem. Be aware of small leaks, and attend to them.
- Attitudes are more important than facts.
- When you get up in the morning you have two choices, to be happy or unhappy. Choose carefully.
- Give yourself a dose of confidence.
- Set yourself goals which you can reach. It is not a good idea to set yourself impossible goals as you will always be disappointed.
- Compare your achievements with your previous ones, not with other people's.
- The mind always tries to achieve what is expected of it.
  Think of failing and you are more likely to fail.
  Think of nothing and your mind will be bored.
  Think of succeeding, and do so.
- Believe in yourself, whatever you are. We all are important to those around us.
- Do whatever job you do as well as you can, for your benefit as well as for society in general.
- Every day do something that you want to do, as opposed to something that you have to do.
- If you tend to do everything yourself, ask for help or give responsibility to others sometimes.
- Consider yourself as well as others. You have needs too, so aim for a good balance.
- Share your feelings and other people's.
- Learn from past mistakes.
- Do not expect to be perfect in the future. Perfection is impossible.

- Aim to be quiet with your own thoughts for part of each day.
- Do not be rushed all day with no time to feel or think.
- Say no sometimes.
- Live in the present more than in the past or in the future.
- Breathe deeply and take a thought vitamin when feeling agitated or impatient, for example in a traffic jam.
- Do not stay in the fast lane of life all the time, or it will go so fast that you will not have time to live it.
- Be a good listener as well as a good talker.
- Compliment others when they deserve it and be happy with them.
- Withdrawal from people and relationships can hurt more than being hurt by them. Reach out to people.
- Anticipate that the best will happen.
- Responsibility is good for you as long as there is neither too much nor too little.
- Continual whining makes problems bigger, not smaller.
- Hope is an excellent bridge.
- With others it is important to be cooperative, but that does not mean that you always give in.
- If no one can help or understand you, you are not communicating.
- Mental pain can be as distressing as physical pain; it is just that others do not see the wound.
- Other people have problems too.
- Think about what you want to do with life. It would be a pity to get to the end and wish you had lived it entirely differently.
- You have a problem? Consider it, read about it, think about it, talk about it. Try going round it, over it, or under it. If all else fails, go right through it, but do not spend your whole life looking at it.
- Worry is an unhealthy, destructive mental habit and an absolute waste of time.
- Never take anxiety or worry to bed with you. They will snore all night.
- Thoughts about situations or people you do not like and cannot change need to be thrown out. We all encounter them, but thinking about them wastes your life and no one else's.

> - Believe in yourself and rebuild your mental immune system with a well-balanced diet of healthy thoughts; then peace, happiness, love, health and humour will smile with you.

THE POWER OF TOUCH

There are many ways of touching.

We can touch with the eyes, silently communicating love, hate, joy, sorrow, pain, fear, uncertainty, etc.

We touch other people with our minds whenever we meet them, and the impression we leave can make them feel better or worse throughout the day. Alternatively, we can make no impression at all and be forgotten in a few minutes. At the other extreme, we may totally alter the other person's life.

The British have always been reserved, shaking hands whilst many other nations use a kiss or embrace. Nowadays, even shaking hands is often replaced by a smile – or a glare. Research has shown, however, that even the mere touching of hands, in passing a letter or stamp for example, creates warmer feelings between people than if they had not touched at all. Other researchers have shown that babies thrive more if touched and cuddled a lot. Elderly people who have lost their life's partner can suffer from a 'touch deficiency' and may benefit from a pet that they can hold and stroke.

Lack of touch can create a lot of mental pain within a family. Misused touch can cause both mental and physical pain. Withdrawal of touch can also easily lead to divorce or unhappiness.

Touch is a way of transferring energy and feelings from one person to another. Touch can cause pleasure or pain, and the immune system responds accordingly.

RELIGION

Religion does not offer an escape into a lifetime of peace and security that can just be soaked up. People who believe in God still have problems, make mistakes and experience pain like everyone else.

A true faith and a good relationship with God can, however, take the di out of distress, while prayer is very efficient at stabilising that inner balance. In the prevention of sickness, as well as in the healing of the body and mind, we have many therapies at our disposal. Faith is one of the great resources available to us all, if we choose to use it.

THE MIND CONNECTION

You communicate with your immune system through your mind. You have your own healing power within, which will work with other forms of medicine.

Every thought, every feeling, every emotion, causes chemicals to be released in the body. It is not difficult to harness this immune power. You do not even need to know the names and actions of all the chemicals. It is simplicity itself. All the good positive and happy thoughts give us a shot of immune- and confidence-boosting chemicals. Dwelling on all the negative ideas, gives us a dose of depressing and suppressing ones. The good news is that you can regulate these shots yourself.

Do not panic when you get a 'negative injection'. We need the negative as well as the positive. A positive attitude to a negative thought is a winner.

Thought is a major weapon in preventing disease and in healing. Today is the first day of the whole of the rest of your life. Why not use this power or, at least, think about it?

26
AGING AND THE IMMUNE SYSTEM

Aging depends not so much on the passage of time as on the result of each individual's biochemical reactions. Barring such things as genetic factors and accidents, it is your body chemistry which determines whether you age quickly or slowly, painfully or beautifully, and the immune system is a key factor in this process.

One theory is that we have a built-in clock and a certain number of cells to use. When those cells are used, that's it. We can make the clock run faster, but probably not slower, and once one body system gives up, the chain reaction starts. The thymus is the master gland of the immune system. The cells of this gland have a more rapid turnover than the cells of any other organ of the body; it must therefore finish first. In fact the thymus goes into decline from the age of puberty – not a time at which you generally consider yourself to be aging.

Another theory is that the older we get, the more toxins we accumulate and the more likely it is that our cells will make genetic errors. If errors occur in body cells, the immune system will not recognise them as self and will attack. If it happens in immune cells, these incorrectly programmed cells could well attack the wrong thing or omit to attack at all – and without an immune system we are merely a feeding ground for any opportunist bugs looking for an easy meal.

IMMUNE CHANGES AS WE AGE

Early in life, in the womb, we potentially have immunocytes to every conceivable antigen, although in practice there are large gaps, because, during the passage of time since man came into being, errors and omissions have been made and passed on. The thymus is very active in the foetus and baby. It switches off all the immunocytes which code for self so that they do not attack anything which belongs to us. Mutator genes are switched on to record alien codes like those of bacteria and viruses. Infant, and particularly foetal, growth is very fast and it is growth hormone which stimulates thymus activity and hence the immune system.

At puberty, sex hormones cause a decrease in the size and activity of the thymus and the mutator genes are switched off. Whatever information our immune cells then have is what they use from then on. The decrease in thymus activity is steep from the age of 12 to 28 years, but the thymus still retains some activity, in that it matures T cells – our T-cell, as opposed to antibody, production remains dependent on the thymus gland throughout life.

Middle age is the crunch time for aging. If we allow the thymus to waste away completely during these middle years, it will not be able to turn off the antibodies and mature T cells properly when mutator genes are switched on again at roughly the end of our reproductive life. It may be easy to see teeth rotting, for example, but not very easy to notice the loss of thymus activity until around the fifth decade, when perhaps viral infections become a problem because of inefficient or insufficient T cells. Antibody production to combat the bacteria which we have encountered before usually remains good in old age, but it is not so reliable for new bugs.

HORMONES AND THE IMMUNE SYSTEM

It used to be thought that the thymus was a redundant organ after about 14 years of age, but we now know that it has a very important function from birth through to death. It is worth looking after it if you wish to retain maximum resistance to disease and to stay as young as you can. We may never discover how to slow aging down, but we can keep it ticking over at its intended rate rather than speeding it up if we look after the immune system.

It is particularly necessary to look after the thymus during the middle years of life. It is stimulated nutritionally by sufficient beta-carotene, vitamin A, zinc, and the amino acids L-ornithine, L-tyrosine, L-tryptophan and glycine, mainly because these nutrients are those which stimulate growth hormone.

Growth hormone production decreases with age and usually stops by the time we are 50 unless we keep it going. Growth hormone, like the sex hormone, oestrogen, can help prevent the mineral depletion from bones that often occurs with aging. Growth hormone is usually released when we exercise, are deprived of food or when we sleep. So good sound sleep, exercise and, for adults, an occasional short fast are beneficial. It should be noted, however, that long-term low-calorie low-nutrient diets do not have a beneficial effect, but instead cause a progressive fall in the basal metabolic rate, such that the whole body slows down. This is why some overweight people who drastically reduce food intake in an attempt to slim, still stay well covered. In slimming it is essential to lose weight slowly and not to disturb the body's chemistry. Putting the body chemistry out is like disturbing the mechanism of an old-fashioned clock – it may never work properly again.

The thyroid hormone, like growth hormone, stimulates the thymus, while corticosteroids, adrenaline and sex hormones suppress it. Strong tea or coffee over-stimulate the adrenals, and so suppress thymus activity.

INDICATORS OF AGING

Amyloid is an eosinophil material comprised partly of insoluble proteins. Lipofuscin is the pigment responsible for the brown age spots; it has a protein component which is highly insoluble and is also an indicator of aging. Collagen is a normal tissue protein and a very reliable indicator of aging. Up to 30 years of age, between 63 per cent and 93 per cent of collagen is soluble and digestible by the enzyme collaginase, but after the age of 60 only 15 per cent to 53 per cent is soluble. Body proteins thus become more insoluble with age. If we keep our protein intake in the moderate rather than the excessive range, and keep it more soluble, we visibly age more slowly than if we eat to excess and form insoluble protein. Vitamin C intake is vital for healthy collagen building, and beta-carotene or vitamin A is also helpful; ensure a good intake of both.

Consequently, as we get older, it is important that we eat the right amount of protein, not too much. Proteins can be made insoluble by the action of free radicals, the action of the latter being a major topic of research on aging and other pathological conditions. Free radicals are formed during many chemical reactions but particularly from utilisation of polyunsaturated fats. We can try to neutralise them by sufficient use of antioxidants, vitamin C being a good antioxidant in our watery parts and vitamin E in our fatty parts. Both promise to be important factors in preventing hastened aging, while high-fat junk-food diets will not provide the necessary antioxidants but will supply an abundance of free radicals.

Vitamin C is vital inside T cells. T cells, remember, contain lysozyme, a deadly enzyme both for germs and also, unfortunately, for our own cells. When the little packets (lysosomes) containing lysozyme are broken, the enzyme destroys the enemy. If there is no enemy, because the T cell got it wrong, or if there is any lysozyme left over, the enzyme can attack us until it is used up (a lot of lysosome activity is thought to be instrumental in lipofuscin pigment formation). Vitamin C provides some protection by mopping up the excess. The level of vitamin C in T cells always goes down with infection. A diet rich in vitamin C will protect against early destruction of the immune system, but smoking causes T cell vitamin C levels to drop.

Folic acid is vital and in animal tests, deficient animals lost 80 per cent of T-cell activity. Women are particularly prone to folate deficiency, and this could be a contributory factor to faster visible aging in women that we would expect in men. Smoking, too, hastens visible aging (wrinkles in particular) considerably.

There is often an increase in serum globulins (the stuff antibodies are made of) with age, but it is probably not an advantage, as many are directed against self. There is also some doubt as to whether this is true aging or merely a disease process, because individuals who were very active, nutrient sufficient and disease free do not appear to get an increase in serum globulins with age.

Atherosclerosis does occur with age to some extent, but arteriosclerosis (hardening of blood vessels) is a diseased state which has only been found in man and whales; hence it is not linked with age, or other animals would get it as they aged too.

Burning ages us, as it causes antibodies to be made to the destroyed tissue protein; hence sunburn ages the skin. Sunburn and free radicals, amongst other things, cause cross-linking and this process makes tissue less elastic and again causes aging. The more cross-linking that occurs, the more sites there are to confuse the immune system. Cross-links are attacked because they are not recognised as self. Ultraviolet B light is a major cause of cross-linking, but it is only a problem around midday; ultraviolet A is less damaging.

We over-consume low-nutrient foods, whereas research has shown time and again in animals that a low-calorie but high-nutrient diet is much more conducive to longevity. The most important regime to follow to avoid premature aging is exactly the opposite to what most people in this country seem to do. Basically we eat too much of too little. It was written on one Egyptian pyramid 5,000 years ago that 'Man lives on a quarter of what he eats. His doctor lives on the remaining three-quarters' – they even over-ate then. Over-eating is a fast method of inducing aging. The poor body, like an overworked sausage factory, tries to process the great quantities of material stuffed in. Often the food lacks the nutrients needed for it to be processed, so the body either has to take these from its structure or not process the food properly. Tubes get blocked, vital materials run out, storage depots overflow. Eventually whichever is the most stressed system, and this varies from body to body, sighs with exhaustion and takes a vacation. If its owner is lucky, the system may be coaxed back into production again; and if not, aging is no longer a problem!

At the other end of the scale, many nutrient deficiencies, too many to mention singly, cause premature aging. Generally speaking, early joint or spinal degeneration signals an individual's deficiency of vitamin C and manganese. Those with osteoporosis have probably had a calcium/magnesium imbalance for years. As you get older, you tend to eat more dairy produce and less nuts and seeds, as these are not compatible with false teeth; hence the calcium intake is often out of balance with the magnesium intake. This is often compounded by lack of appropriate exercise.

The right sort of exercise is needed to prevent bone loss. Swimming, whilst being a good exercise for heart, lungs and muscles, is no good for bones. Bones need load-bearing movement and gravity; astronauts suffer from bone loss. So walking is an excellent activity for people wishing to keep their bones. Calcium is lost from bones even during sleep, so it is wise to do exercises if having to endure bed rest for any period of time.

A lack of growth and sex hormones exacerbate the problem, which is why many women suffer from osteoporosis after menopause. Smoking increases the rate of bone thinning considerably, as do prolonged low-calorie low-nutrient diets or very high-protein diets. Frequent use of antacids will also increase the risk as stomach acid is needed for calcium absorption. Children absorb most of the calcium in their food, but adults absorb usually less than 50 per cent. With age, stomach acid production decreases and hence absorption of many vital nutrients is impaired. This is often due to eating and drinking hot food over a lifetime. What is your stomach, after all, but a piece of meat? Continually bathe it in hot tea, coffee, soup, etc., and what do you have but a denatured cooked stomach, no longer able to perform as well as when it was raw.

Whilst calcium comes out of the bones with age, it seems to go into other tissues, like the brain, arteries, kidneys and heart and this may lead to the calcium forming a gel/or solidifying in these areas. We need to stay as fluid as possible; hardening of attitudes, arteries, joints, and tissues causes us to slow down and to seize up.

IMMUNE POWER

In youth or even in middle age, it is easy to shrug off old age till later. However, you and your body are a life-long partnership and there is no getting away from it. Some day, old age will be the present and will to some extent be as beautiful or as painful as your previous lifestyle has made it. A body can serve reliably and actively if it is looked after, allowing you to enjoy a happy, healthy retirement.

We sometimes need help with keeping our body in balance or with restoring it to health if it has gone wrong, and call upon a physician, who is a person skilled in the art of healing. By physician, we usually mean a doctor of medicine, because modern medicine has developed many skills to prevent disease and repair damaged bodies; we all need the help of such a person at some time during our lives.

There are other physicians whose knowledge can be helpful in enabling us to stay in optimum health. Psychiatrists, psychologists and various counsellors can help us to heal the mind. Nutritionists can correct the body's nutrient intake and so help us to make and mend more effectively. There are homoeopaths, herbalists, osteopaths, physiotherapists, those who teach sport and movement, relaxation and meditation, and a whole host of others whose therapies will improve our health. We may call on God, the Physician, to help us deal with the legion of mental, physical, emotional and spiritual viruses that try to invade us.

There is, however, another medical team who are usually forgotten and neglected, although always on call. These physicians work, regardless of race, colour, belief, wealth, power or deeds, constantly striving to save our lives, whether we help or hinder them. This team, skilled in the art of healing, is the immune army.

There is no doubt that the immune system is affected by our diet, our lifestyle, our thoughts, our movements and our environment. The good news is that by taking care of and improving all these things, we can undoubtedly improve our health. Whatever we have now can be better and stronger if we cooperate with this immune army.

Whether trying to prevent or needing to cure any illness, we should consider the advice of all of our physicians, but help from outside is only part of the treatment; in the final analysis, it is up to us to heal ourselves with our own immune power.

INDEX

All Optima books are available at your bookshop or newsagent, or can be ordered from the following address:

Optima, Cash Sales Department,
PO Box 11, Falmouth, Cornwall TR10 9EN

Please send cheque or postal (no currency), and allow 60p for postage and packing for the first book, plus 25p for the second book and 15p for each additional book ordered up to a maximum charge of £1.90 in the UK.

Customers in Eire and BFPO please allow 60p for the first book, 25p for the second book plus 15p per copy for the next 7 books, thereafter 9p per book.

Overseas customers please allow £1.25 for postage and packing for the first book and 28p per copy for each additional book.